Awareness

A Path To
Spiritual And Physical
Health And Well-Being

Glenn Molinari

Awareness - A Path To Spiritual And Physical Health And Well-Being

Copyright © 2014 by Glenn Molinari

Updated January, 2018 (Chakra graphic added)

Glenn Molinari

P.O. Box 1534

Cornville, AZ 86325

Library of Congress

Awareness - A Path To Spiritual And Physical Health And Well-Being

/ Glenn Molinari

Registration Number: TXu 001918151 / 2014-03-10

Publisher: Glenn Molinari

ISBN: 978-0-9854784-4-5

Also available as an eBook at online retailers

Preface

This book presents information to increase awareness of:

Ways to nurture and take care of the physical body

Ways to strengthen your connection to Spirit

How to recognize when you are accessing and sharing Love
or something other than Love.

It includes information on commonly unknown aspects of:

Dental problems and their systemic affects

GMO Foods

Xenohormones from the environment and foods

Prenatal Trauma

Vanishing twins

Receiving your own guidance

Recognizing the source as Love or anything else

Healing vs. curing

Releasing negative *feelings*, emotions and memories

The importance of the subconscious mind

I recommend reading the Glossary before reading the rest of the book..

I use the book and the processes as the basis for my own personal clearing and healing.

I have listed Sources of Information and Sources that lead me to further awareness, intuition and knowing.

You can confirm and expand on the information presented by your own research as you choose.

I have minimized use of the word *not* except for a few instances where the original source used the word or for simplicity These are underlined and bold to bring the use to awareness. I have done the same for the word *but*. It is amazing how often we use these words without even realizing it.

Glenn Molinari

FREE downloadable and printable PDFs of the meditations, exercises and prayers in this book are available at   http://www.twochoices.net/FREE_PDFs.html

They do not include the explanations and information in the book, so I suggest you read the book first.

Acknowledgements

Thanks to all those who have allowed me to share and fine tune this.

Special Thanks to Jewels Maloney.

She was instrumental in helping me with the references, shared some important formatting tips and helped to fine tune the wording.

Dr. Maloney may be reached at:

http://Ascensionisnow.com

Table of Contents

Preface

Acknowledgements

Introduction and Making Choices vi

Glossary vii

Chapter 1   Physical And Medical

    Holistic Medicine and Dentistry 1

    Dental And Mouth 6

        Mercury Toxicity - Overview 6

        Mercury Amalgam Fillings - How Safe Are They 6

        History Of Mercury Amalgam In Fillings 7

        Banning Mercury In Amalgam Fillings and
        How The American Dental Association Was Formed ... 8

        Why Eliminate the use of Amalgam (mercury) Fillings? ... 9

        Should You Consider Having Your Amalgam Fillings
        Removed? 10

        Removing Mercury Amalgam Fillings, Mercury Toxicity And
        Chronic Health Issues 11

        Holistic Vs. Conventional Dentistry 12

        Tooth To Organs And Emotions Chart 15

        Cavitations 21

    Nutrition

        The Basics 22

        Phytates 24

        Thiocyanate 25

        Oxalic Acid 26

        Purine 26

        Soy As An Enzyme Inhibitor 28

        Other Things Some People May Want To Be Aware Of ... 29

	Water	29
	Heirloom Seeds	30
	Hybrid Plants And Animals	31
GMO Foods, Herbicides, Animal Feed Additives		
	What Are GMO Foods?	32
	GMO Is No Longer Just For Foods (sometimes called GE)	32
	Bt-toxin Produced In GM Corn And Cotton Plants	34
	Glyphosate Toxicity—Another Hidden Danger Of GE Foods	35
	Common GMO Foods	38
	GMO Companies	40
	Genetically Modified Soil Fungus And Algae As Nutritional Supplements In Organic Food (including baby formula)	42
	Livestock And Animal Feed Additives	44
	Ractopamine (Animal Feed Additive)	45
	Zilmax (Cattle Feed Additive)	46
	Glyphosate Contamination (Active Ingredient in Herbicides)	47
	rBGH Hormones (To Increase Milk Production In Cows)	49
	Mutagenesis (An Unregulated Form Of Genetic Modification)	51
Poisons And Toxins		52
Xenohormones And Estrogen Dominance		53
Ideal Nutrition		61
Chapter 2	Daily Practices	
	Upgrade Internal Dialog And Verbal Communication	63
	Words To Avoid Using	63
	The Word 'Should' And The Inner Critic	64
	Speaking, Communicating And Doing Your Best	65
Chapter 3	What Is Man	67
Chapter 4	Balance And The Nature Of Duality	69
Chapter 5	The Importance of the Subconscious and How To Strengthen Your Connection With LOVE	71

Chapter 6   Channels, Mediums, False Information And Prophecies

    Definitions Of Channel, Channeling And Flow   77

    Receiving Your Own Guidance   78

    What Is Distortion?   How Is It Recognized?   78

    Knowing When The Source Is Communicating Truth   79

    Prophecy   79

    Subjugation   80

Chapter 7   Knowing, *Feeling*, Awareness And Judgment

    What Is "Knowing" And What Is " Being Fully Aware"   81

    Difference Between Awareness , Knowing And Judgment   82

    How To Recognize When You Are Sliding From Awareness Into Judgment   83

    Wisdom and Power   84

    There Is Only Light   88

Chapter 8   Desires, Programs And Who Is In Charge

    You Create Your Own Fate   89

    Who Is In Charge?   91

    Naming Stars And Planets And Dogma   93

    Planets, Astrology and Mans Thoughts   94

    Too Much Information   95

    Information Compressed In The Form Of *Feelings*   96

Chapter 9   Healing, Curing And Knowing When To Step Back

    Healing Vs. Curing   99

    Helping When It Is Against Natural Universal Laws   100

    Healing the Past, Present And Future - Explanation And Charts   102

Chapter 10   Receiving Your Own Information and Guidance Through *Feeling*

    Practice *Feeling*   105

Chapter 11   Life Long Effects Of Prenatal And Perinatal Experiences
             (Including Toxins) And Vanishing Twins

             Introduction To Information On Prenates And Vanishing Twins   107

             The Vulnerable Prenate (Unborn Child) And Its Effects On Later   108
             Life

             Vanishing Twins And Its Effects On Later Life   119

Chapter 12   Five Methods of Healing, Clearing and Releasing   127

             1) Through Prayer   129

             2) Affirmations   129

             3) 'Memories Replaying' - Erasing The Energetic Attachment To   130
             And *Feelings* From

             4) Releasing Trapped *Feelings*/Emotions Based On Bradley
             Nelsons' "The Emotion Code"

             Explanation Of "The Emotion Code"   131

             Six Kinds Of Imbalance - Basic Explanations   134

                   1) Infections And Infestations In Detail   136

                   2) Structural Misalignments In Detail   137

                   3) Nutritional Deficiencies In Detail   138

                   4) Toxins And Poisons In Detail   139

                   5) Energy Field Imbalances In Detail   139

                   6) Trapped *Feelings* And Emotions In Detail   140

             The Heart Wall   142

             Magnetism And Using Magnets To Release Trapped *Feelings*   143
             And Emotions

             Which Magnets To Use   145

             Using The Emotion Code   146

             'Soul Echoes' and The Emotion Codd   147

                   The Actual Process - Glenn's Flow Chart   149

                   The Actual Process - Bradley Nelson's Emotions Chart   150

5) Clearing Suppressed *Feelings*/Emotions Based on John Ruskan's *"Emotional Clearing Process"*

    Introduction To John Ruskan's *"Emotional Clearing Process"*   151

    The Truth About 'The Law of Attraction   152

    Emotions And Addictions   153

    Further Explanation   155

        How It Works   159

        The Process Of Entering The Witness   165

    Activating Healing Energy by 'Entering The Witness'
    The Actual Process   166

Chapter 13   Self Reflection and Questions To Ask Yourself

    The Importance Of The Subconscious Mind As A Key   169

    1 -   Worthiness   170

    2 -   Reclaim Your Will   172

    3 -   Energize Your Body   174

    4 -   Money and Abundance   176

    5 -   Tame Your Mind   177

    6 -   Trust Your Intuition   178

    7 -   Accept Your *Feelings* and Emotions   180

    8 -   Face Your Fears   184

    9 -   Illuminate Your Shadow   186

    10 - Sexuality and Sensuality   190

    11 - Awaken and Open Your Heart   192

    12 - Serve Your World and Your Self   193

    Other Thoughts To Ponder   194

Chapter 14   Tools, Crutches and Traps   195

Suggested Reading And Web Sites   197

References   199

About Glenn   202

Contact Glenn   202

Introduction

I gathered the information included here for myself and others beginning in the late 1980s. It is from various sources. I included the source information where I still have it. I strongly believe this information to be correct.

The first chapter is about physical well being. It has information I have found valid and helpful for myself. I believe that connecting more closely to Great Spirit and LOVE also requires taking care of the physical body. I am still far from perfect in my eating habits and life style and yet I have noticed I am doing better as I continue my journey.

Like physical healing, when you do Spiritual house clearing, your physical body can have reactions or go through detoxing symptoms. As with *any* type of healing, when you are detoxing, whether it be physical, mental, emotional or Spiritual you may have symptoms of the detox.

Great Spirit and Great Spirit's Helpers know what is best and what you can handle. Prior to healing you may ask Great Spirit and Great Spirit's Helpers as are best to make it gentle enough so you can continue your daily responsibilities.

You may have disorientation, vertigo, emotional release (unpleasant *feelings*/emotions, unpleasant dreams) while healing. This is often the case with any healing, including the use of such things as Flower Essences, Reiki, Shamanistic Practices, Soul Retrieval, Inner Child Healing, Prayer, Fasting and The Use of Antibiotics.

Allow the release and thank what is coming to the surface to be healed, erased, forgiven and loved (an emotion, *feeling*, thought, physical detox, etc).

You may get very tired for a few hours or for several days. If so, rest when your schedule permits.

You may perspire a lot, get rashes/hives, urinate a lot, vomit, and/or have many loose bowel movements. This is the body eliminating physical and non-physical (emotions, *feelings*, thoughts) toxins.

NOTE: You may see immediate results or it may take a while before you see any changes in your life, awareness and health. Divinity knows what layers and what toxins need to be healed, erased, forgiven and loved. Divinity also knows the order in which to process them and the timing for each.

As you heal be careful as you reduce or even eliminate traditional therapies. If you are on prescription medicines consult with your doctor before discontinuing. As an example, blood pressure medicine can often be reduced or eliminated as you manage your weight, eat healthier and learn to reduce stress.

Glossary

Man (capitalized): A manifestation of ' eternal Mind'. *Thinking, intelligent beings* (Bibliography Translator's preface in "*Anastasia*", book 1)

human being: This term has a problem in that it suggests a formation of the species from matter, or earth.

Humus - the organic constituent of soil is associated with lowly concepts, such as *humble and humility*. Also, the word *human* is essentially an adjective, even though commonly used as a noun in today's English. (Bibliography Translator's preface in "*Anastasia*", Book 1)

man (lower case): Adult male human

woman (lower case): Adult female human

Destiny Tunnel: Moment to moment, as you and others make choices, the "Destiny Tunnel" shifts and changes the future and past, as well as the present. Without conscious thought and conscious healing, 99% of possible "Time Lines" lead to the same basic outcome. It takes conscious choices to shift.

Prayer: Prayer is basically a sincere attempt to communicate with Source and the Divine within yourself. The key is to be present, authentic and sincere with LOVE in your heart. Practice your own prayers instead of repeating others' words from memory. It often seems that when most people pray they are asking for things and Divine Intervention rather than giving thanks and asking for guidance. Examples of what I believe are powerful and positive prayers are in Chapter 7 of my first book, *Two Choices - Divine Love Or Anything Else.*

Affirmations: Affirmations are often described as positive statements. They are used to retrain the subconscious mind and create constructive changes in yourself and the physical world. Every thought and word is an affirmation. All of our inner dialogues are streams of affirmations. Saying and thinking positive affirmations will shift you from the negative to the positive. Each negative thought and word will create more of the negative. Affirmations are effective on the level of the subconscious mind and are very powerful. Avoiding the use of the words *not, but, need to, try, want to, should* and *could* is critical in affirmations. Realize *don't, won't, can't* and *shouldn't* are all "not" words. If there are negative and/or limiting *feelings*, emotions, memories or beliefs involved, the effectiveness of positive affirmations <u>may</u> be limited until the *feelings*, emotions, memories replaying or beliefs involved are cleared and healed. Sometimes the affirmation itself created the healing.

Memories Replaying: Memories replaying, like old tapes from past experiences, keep negative and limiting beliefs energized. For example, one might delete an email, however, until the 'deleted' folder is emptied and the email is permanently trashed the email is still there and so is the message.

***Feelings* and Emotions:** There is such a fine line between the definitions of '*feeling*' 'and emotion' that they can be easily confused. In many dictionaries one word is used to define the other. I understand *feelings* as held inside and often unexpressed, and emotions as expressed *feelings*, both verbally and nonverbally. As an example, if you *feel* angry at someone **but** put on a happy face, that is a *feeling*. If you express the *feeling* outwardly that is an emotion. An emotion is the outward expression of a *feeling*. This is how I use the words in this book. F*eelings* and emotions are healed and released in the same way.

Limiting and Negative Beliefs: Negative and limiting/interfering beliefs are always caused by and energized by trapped, suppressed, repressed, unresolved *feelings* and emotions and/or by memories replaying. Even if a belief is cleared, it may be re-energized unless the underlying *feeling*, emotion or memory replaying has been healed and released. The belief is often healed by healing and transmuting the *feelings*, emotions and memories replaying that energized it. If the negative/limiting belief remains after the *feelings*, emotions and memories replaying have been healed, transmuted and released, the belief itself can then be cleared.

Akashic Records: Is a term used for all the "records" or information of the past, the present and the future. This includes all Man's thoughts and actions and their consequences. This is beyond just human thoughts and actions and includes the thoughts and actions of all manifestations of Man ('Eternal Mind' -'*Thinking, intelligent beings'*). They als*o* include all the infinite potential possibilities in 'All That Is". We all have the ability to access these records without the need of an intermediary, guru, sage, psychic or medium. We can chose to access them through LOVE or through 'Anything Else'. With practice you will be able to access them more and more clearly. It is important to be discerning when accessing them. The records are in constant flux since there are always new thoughts and actions being added. The past, the present and the future are changeable with LOVE and with fear. Change them with LOVE.

Honor:
Dictionary definitions:

> mark of respect; mark of distinction; tribute; pay homage to; personal dignity that sometimes leads to recognition and glory.

Reasons to be careful with this word.

> When you say to someone, "I am honored" or when someone says to you, "I am honored", it is easy to place the person being addressed as a superior. We are all equally special in our own unique ways. I prefer saying, "I am thankful", or, "I am grateful" to avoid pedestals and *feelings* of superiority or inferiority.

Work

"Work", when doing healing 'work', includes healing, releasing, relinquishing, 'letting go', clearing and transmuting. It only includes 'curing' of physical symptoms and ailments if they are no longer needed for soul growth and spiritual development. If you are working on physical, emotional or mental symptoms make sure you remember the previous sentence. Keep enjoyment in the process.

Even though the Unihipili (see Chapter 4) is much more powerful than the conscious mind, it is in many ways like a three or four year old child. It needs guidance and LOVE. It also likes to investigate. The Unihipili, or child within, will respond or react according to your "choice". The Unihipili, like children, dislikes work and likes to play, therefore I use the word *work* carefully when doing any kind of healing, releasing and transmuting.

Healing, Transmuting, Releasing and Integrating:

Any time any form of the words *heal, clear* or *release* is used in a clearing or healing it includes the process of healing the energetic causes, transmuting any 'negative' into its 'positive' and Loving counterpart, releasing the unhealthy attachments and integrating the positive, life affirming and Loving aspects into yourself. If you have a pain, discomfort, injury or disease treat it at the physical level with physical means. It is always a good idea to also treat the pain, discomfort, injury or disease by Healing, Transmuting, Releasing and Integrating at the spiritual, mental and emotional levels as well.

Transmutation:

The dictionary definition is change/alteration/ transformation/metamorphosis. As used in this book, transmutation is one of Divinity's tools for changing what is often referred to as dark/negative/evil into LOVE and LIGHT.

"As is best":

Many of my prayers, the way I say them, are finished with "as is best". This is my way of turning the prayer or request over to Great Spirit/God/Divinity without attachment to a desired outcome or an expectation. If you have another way of turning it over to Great Spirit use your way. Just make sure you turn it over. Also, remember you are responsible to do your part. If you sit on the couch and eat or drink all day and pray, "make me healthy" or "make me wealthy", do you really expect to be made healthy or wealthy.

Co-Creation and Manifesting:

To me there is a difference between 'co-creation' with Great Spirit and 'manifestation'. Co-creation is more at the spiritual and energetic level and Manifestation is more at the physical and human action level.

Judgment and Nonjudgmental:

I use 'non-judgmental' as meaning **allowing** the other person or Being their own path, free will, truths and perceptions. Any time you are judging, you are in some way judging your self. A decision based on an objective observation is different than a 'judgment' and more like assessment. With objective assessment you can then take the appropriate action or inaction.

Accept and Accepting:

Rather than using the word non-judgmental, it is more potent, more clear and more uplifting to say "unconditionally accepting" or "unconditional acceptance". This is at spiritual and energetic levels to allow others their own perceptions, choices and realities. It is appropriate and wise to protect yourself from any kind of abuse or mistreatment, whether verbal, physical or very subtle. If someone or an organization is abusing or mistreating you in anyway, distance yourself from them energetically **and** physically if you are able. If you are **temporarily** in a position where you are physically 'trapped', use a method to prevent taking on the energy as a personal belief. Acceptance is different than accepting negative people or circumstances into your life. It refers primarily to your *feelings*, as they are, relative to the negative people or circumstances. See Yourself as safe.

Remember to unconditionally accept your self.

Compassion - As We Have Been Taught By Society And The Dictionary:

sorrow for the sufferings or trouble of another or others, with the urge to help; pity; deep sympathy; the feeling of empathy for others; emotion that we feel in response to the suffering of others that motivates a desire to help; suffering together with another; participation in suffering; requires walking with the other person and feeling with them their suffering; deep awareness of the suffering of another coupled with the wish to relieve it. This version of compassion defines someone as a victim and is thus a form of judgment.

Compassion - Higher Dimensional Version Of:

Deep awareness of the suffering of another without the need to relieve it, *feeling* total appreciation for its value; a state of unconditional acceptance and LOVE.

Accept that each person is choosing their problem(s) and have to connect with their own Higher SELF in order to heal;

We must shift our perspective of compassion and begin using a version that is beyond what we have been taught. We must move into the realm of unconditional acceptance, leaving pity and the need to 'fix' behind.

We must suspend all judgment of the actions of another. We must be aware of those actions, how painful they are and at the same time realize that they have a value and that this value pertains to the role they play in facilitating our spiritual growth as souls

Power - Dictionary Definition:

Authority, control, influence, supremacy, command, dominance, force.

Manipulation would be the key word; the power to manipulate situations and those around you.

Power - As Used In This Book:

Personal power comes from wisdom. Real personal power is a subtle quality of Beingness rather than a force.

Real power has nothing to do with control, especially the control of others. Conversely, real power is surrendering to the highest good. Real power naturally settles within one's Beingness of its own accord as Wisdom and Love increase.

Wisdom - Dictionary Definition:

Understanding, knowledge, intelligence, accumulated learning, opinion widely held, accumulated philosophic or scientific learning, the judicious application of knowledge.

Wisdom - As Used In This Book

Wisdom has nothing to do with the level of one's attained knowledge, age, intelligence or I.Q. rating. Wisdom is born of LOVE arising from the heart. Wisdom becomes part of your Being.

Some aspects of wisdom: Acceptance, Patience and Perseverance, Attitude, Silence, Personal Responsibility, Gentleness and Serenity, Value, Priorities and Respect

True Wisdom is beyond words and the intellect, and is only fully understood by the heart through Awareness.

To understand wisdom as clearly as possible with the intellect, the main aspects of wisdom also need to be understood. These are expanded on in chapter 6.

"Amen" at the end of prayers

How many of us have said the word "Amen" at the end of a prayer without really giving it a second thought? Have you ever said "Amen" , without thought, as a ratification of what is said? You may be saying, "May it be done as the speaker has prayed". Did you fully understand the prayer and did you fully agree with it?

As regards the etymology, which is the study of the origins of words, many believe "Amen" is a derivative from the Hebrew verb *aman* "to strengthen" or "confirm". Some believe the word was originally derived from a Sanskrit word "aum", meaning "to sound out loudly" and some believe it simply means "truly" or "so be it". Is it simply a form of affirmation or confirmation of the speaker's own thought?

In forms of worship a final amen, as now used, often sums up and confirms a prayer.

In many cases the word "Amen" is used as nothing more than a formula of conclusion — *finis,* indicating that the statement or prayer is ended and completed.

The seeming ambiguity of the word "Amen" is why I finish my prayers with "As is best" and "Thank you".

Unihipili: *(u·hi·ni·pi·li)*

The Hawaiian name for what is sometimes called the subconscious/inner/emotional/intuitive mind.

I prefer the Hawaiian name, Unihipili, for the subconscious mind. There is nothing sub about the subconscious mind. It is more in touch with 'Reality' than the conscious mind. It may be lost and need guidance from the conscious mind to connect to LOVE, and once it is it will help the conscious mind and all aspects of you connect more strongly to LOVE also.

The Unihipili (subconscious) or child within will respond or react according to your "choice." This child within is different than "the inner child" as used in inner child healing and soul retrieval. "The inner child" (or children) are a part of the Unihipili.

It is extremely important to let the Unihipili know it is loved and to teach it and your conscious mind to communicate with each other and the Divine.

A simple and fast way to begin gaining the trust and support of your Unihipili is in my first book, *Two Choices - Divine Love Or Anything Else* and in Chapter 5 of this book.

'Brain' and 'Mind'

There is a difference between 'brain' and 'mind'. Our brain is a physical part of our physical body. Our mind is much more. Our brain does have two hemispheres. The left brain deals with logic and data and the right brain deals with *feeling*s, emotions and intuition. This is an oversimplification and some processes spread across the divide. The right brain is the part of the brain that connects with mind. Mind may be unlimited

Even though these are 'my' definitions, I hope they are thought-provoking for you. Think for yourself.

Chapter 1
Physical And Medical

Before reading the rest of the book I strongly suggest to read the glossary. This will help to clarify my use of certain terms and words and allow you to reword as you wish when I use those terms.

Holistic Medicine And Dentistry

The holistic concept unifies the domains of body, mind and spirit. Holistic Medicine is making inroads into our consciousness that were lost as we came to rely almost entirely on our intellectual powers of observation, analysis and deduction. Perhaps it was our conscious, intellectual mind that separated them and made the body primary.

It is unfortunate that there seems to be barriers and a lack of cooperation and respect between the schools of medicine. It seems that many of these systems are devoted to defending their individual orthodoxies rather than being devoted to determining the best treatment for individual patients. They can, and sometimes do, work together to effect the maximal health outcomes for each individual. It will be great when there is an open exchange of each other's principles and true communication and acceptance of the best of each disciplines treatment paradigms. That will be truly Holistic and Integrative.

Some Of The More Common Types Of Medicine Practices

Allopathy (modern western medicine)

This is the least holistic medical practice and relies almost entirely on our intellectual powers of observation, analysis and deduction. It is appropriate for broken bones, severe injury and other 'physical' problems. It may be the least effective form of medicine for treating the underlying causes of disease and a true 'healing'. It is best to treat the underlying cause using an holistic approach as well treating symptoms using the allopathic method.

Allopathic refers to mainstream medical use of pharmacologically active agents or physical interventions to **treat or suppress symptoms** or pathophysiolic processes of diseases or conditions. The expression was coined in 1810 by the creator of homeopathy, Samuel Hahnemann (1755–1843). In such circles, the expression "allopathic medicine" is still used to refer to "the broad category of medical practice that is sometimes called Western Medicine or Modern Medicine"

There is also allopathic (conventional) and holistic dentistry as explained later in this chapter.

Homeopathy

The principle of treating "like with like" dates back to Hippocrates (460-377BC). In its current form, homeopathy has been widely used worldwide for more than 200 years.

It was discovered by a German doctor, Samuel Hahnemann, who, shocked with the harsh medical practices of the day (which included blood-letting, purging and the use of poisons such as arsenic), looked for a way to reduce the damaging side-effects associated with medical treatment.

He began experimenting on himself and a group of healthy volunteers, giving smaller and smaller medicinal doses, and found that as well as reducing toxicity, the medicines actually appeared to be more effective in lower doses. He also observed that symptoms caused by toxic 'medicines' such as mercury, were similar to those of the diseases they were being used to treat; example - syphilis, which lead to the principle he described as 'like cures like'.

Hahnemann went on to document his work, and his texts formed the foundations of homeopathic medicine as it is practiced today. A BBC Radio 4 documentary aired in December 2010 described Hahnemann as a medical pioneer who worked tirelessly to improve medical practice, insisting that medicines were tested before use.

Osteopathy

D.O.s are trained and licensed to examine patients, prescribe medicine and perform surgery like an M.D. To become a doctor of osteopathy, one must complete four years of undergraduate work, usually in a science field, followed by four years of medical school. D.O.s complete an extra 300 to 500 hours studying the body's musculoskeletal system and learn hands-on methods of diagnosis and treatment. D.O.s are licensed by the region in which they live, and in many areas can become board certified after a two to six year residency and completion of board certification exams. D.O.s can also choose to specialize in a particular field, as M.D.s do.

A doctor of osteopathy is trained to palpate, or to *feel* out what is sometimes called the body's living anatomy. The D.O. is concerned with how fluids flow throughout the body, the texture and movement of tissues, and the structure of the body. The emphasis is on the musculoskeletal system, which is the body's system of nerves, muscles, and bones. A doctor of osteopathy attempts to determine how disease or injury to one particular system or body part affects another.

Many D.O.s use a technique called **Osteopathic Manipulative Treatment** (OMT) in addition to traditional medicines and treatments to treat their patients. They believe that stress and posture can affect the systems of the body and hinder their proper functions, thus causing disease and illness. Through OMT, they manipulate the body in certain ways to assist it in utilizing its natural healing system freely, with no hindrances. If the body is in the correct position, it can work to heal itself. D.O.s can release bones and joints that have become compressed, thereby affecting other systems.

Chiropractic (alignment of skeletal vertebrae to improve nervous system function)

No part of your body escapes the dominance of your nervous system. Improper function of the spine due to slight misalignments—called subluxations—can cause poor health or function, even in areas far removed from the spine and spinal cord itself. Misalignments can also reduce the ability of your body to adapt to its ever-changing environment. Even the slightest malfunction of your spine may alter the regular transmission of nerve impulses, preventing the associated portion of your body from responding optimally.

Chiropractic is a natural form of health care that uses spinal adjustments to correct these misalignments and restore proper function to the nervous system, helping your body to heal naturally. Chiropractic does**n't** use drugs or surgery. Rather, a chiropractic spinal adjustment—the application of a precise force to a specific part of the spinal segment—corrects the misalignment, permitting normal nerve transmission and assisting your body to recuperate on its own.

Herbology (use of herbal medicines)

Medicinally, an herb is any plant part or plant used for its therapeutic value. Many of the world's herbal traditions also include mineral and animal substances as "herbal medicines.

Herbal medicine is the art and science of using herbs for promoting health and preventing and treating illness. It has persisted as the world's primary form of medicine since the beginning of time, with a written history more than 5000 years old. While the use of herbs in America has been overshadowed by dependence on modern medications the last 100 years, 75% of the world's population still rely primarily upon traditional healing practices, most of which is herbal medicine.

Most pharmaceutical drugs are single chemical entities that are highly refined and purified and are often synthesized in a lab. In 1987 about 85% of modern drugs were originally derived from plants. Currently, only about 15% of drugs are derived from plants. In contrast, herbal medicines are prepared from living or dried plants and contain hundreds to thousands of interrelated compounds. Science is beginning to demonstrate that the safety and effectiveness of herbs is often related to the synergy of its many constituents.

The primary focus of the herbalist is to treat people as individuals irrespective of the disease or condition they have and to stimulate their innate healing power through the use of such interventions as herbs, diet and lifestyle. The primary focus of conventional physicians is to attack diseases using strong chemicals that are difficult for the body to process, or through the removal of organs. This focus ignores the unique makeup of the individual and many patients under conventional care suffer from side effects that are as bad as the condition being treated. The philosophical difference between herbalists and conventional physicians has profound significance.

Naturopathy (probably the most holistic.)

A Naturopath is a health practitioner who applies natural therapies. Her/his spectrum comprises far more than fasting, nutrition, water, and exercise; it includes approved natural healing practices such as Homeopathy, Acupuncture, and Herbal Medicine, as well as the use of modern methods like Bio-Resonance, Ozone-Therapy, and Colon Hydrotherapy. At a time when modern technology, environmental pollution, poor diet, and stress play a significant role in the degradation of health, a Naturopath's ability to apply natural methods of healing is of considerable importance. Frequently, a Naturopath is the last resort in a patient's long search for health. Providing personalized care to each patient, the naturopath sees humankind as a holistic unity of body, mind, and spirit.

Ayurvedic

Inherent in Ayurvedic principles is the concept that you are capable of taking charge of your own life and healing.

More than simply medical care, Ayurvedic offers a philosophy whereby one may prevent unnecessary suffering and live a long, healthy life. Known as the mother of all medical systems, Ayurveda has undergone continuous research, development and refinement over the past 5,000 years. Originally from India, Ayurveda is currently experiencing world-wide popularity as a revival sweeps in all continents. Ayurveda employs the judicious application of nutritional guidance, herbal medicines, exercise therapy, transcendental meditation and many special rejuvenation and purification therapies. Preferring to focus on the type of person who has the disease, rather than just understanding the type of disease the person has, Ayurveda is a patient-orientated system of healing.

Dentistry

Only recently has the field of dentistry been let back into the "health field" with the recent scientific validation of the "links" between dental infection (gum disease , root canal infections) and the chronic systemic diseases that are the bane of modern life, including cardiovascular disease (heart attacks and strokes) and diabetes.

If the mind and brain powerfully affect the spirit then the brain and central nervous system function should be included in the Holistic Health Paradigm. There is a powerful structural component that influences the function of the brain and the balance in the nervous system that is woefully unknown. It occurs at the intersection of dentistry and osteopathic medicine.

Intersection Of Dentistry And Osteopathic Medicine

There is a connection between stress and health. A little stress stimulates the body, mind, and spirit; too much overwhelms the nervous system and causes disease (dis-ease). Excess stress of any kind; psychological, emotional, chemical, nutritional or physical, causes the nervous system to become dysfunctional. There needs to be a balance between the sympathetic (flight or fight reaction) and the parasympathetic (rest, relax, digest, heal) sides of the autonomic (automatic) nervous system. Research has now clearly shown that dysfunction in the human jaw joints and/or their muscles (TMJ, TMD) create the same reactions in the body as other forms of stress. Unlike other forms of stress which usually are limited by time, TMJ Dysfunction is usually permanent unless treated by an unusual dentist who understands the unique function of this unique joint.

A little stress has a positive influence for the organism. A permanent or chronic stress causes deterioration in Thymus function (master gland of immune system), exhaustion of the Adrenals (stress glands) and micro bleeding in the intestinal tract. Overall this creates an increase in the inflammatory index of the whole human body. An increase of the body's inflammatory index is related to our modern diseases of heart attacks, strokes, arthritis, diabetes and others.

The TMJs are also related to function of the Cranio-Sacral system according to the Cranial Osteopathic Physicians who study the structure, health and function of the brain and the rest the central nervous system. This includes the dural membrane and the spinal cord. It turns out the human skull is actually slightly flexible. It needs to be flexible because the brain expands and contracts about 10-12 times per minute (You may have observed this undulating pattern in the soft spot of a 1 month old bald headed infant).

The brain expands and contracts because it produces and pumps the Cerebral Spinal Fluid that surrounds and supports the brain and the spinal cord physically. The cranium (skull) is flexible because of the way the skull bones fit together to become hinged joints capable of this almost imperceptible movement. If the bone's joints (sutures) are out of place the skull loses its flexibility which can create pressure on the brain. In addition, as the skull bones are tweaked out of alignment it pulls on the dural membrane (dura mater - which means tough membrane) which encapsulates the brain and spinal cord. This then relays the misalignment to the top three neck vertebra and then to the top of the sacral bone to which the hip bones join. Therefore, bite discrepancies caused by crooked teeth, poorly designed fillings and crowns, and misaligned jaws (TMD) can also cause misalignment in the neck, back or hips. This is often the cause of neck, back and hip pain. Most headaches have a component of bite discrepancy to them. This interference causing dysfunction within the Cranio-sacral system may be the reason that TMJ problems cause so much distress in the human body.

In a practical sense this means those of you with headaches, back, hip and leg pain who are unable to find relief with medicine or physical modalities and Chiropractic may need to find a dentist trained in TMJ therapy and cranio-sacral function. Why? To help out your brain and improve your "body, mind and spirit".

Nutrition is arguably the worst insult to our health in these United States. Poor nutrition, beginning in the womb, is the major cause of bad bites. Familiarize yourself with the substantial damage that poor food quality inflicts on the human race.

Poor nutrition leads to physical and physiological dysfunction. The increase of nutritionally induced allergies leads to mouth breathing in the majority of our infants; which leads to chronic poor tongue posture (because we have to breathe through our mouths); which leads to orthodontic problems, TMJ problems and then in middle age to snoring and sleep apnea problems due to the inadequate airways that were never developed properly.

If you snore, especially if you snore loudly and are experiencing daytime fatigue, talk to your primary care doctor or sleep physician soon.

Dental And Mouth

This section is included because I firmly believe that problems in the mouth can have systemic and even catastrophic effects on the body.

Traditional Asian medicine has long maintained that every body part (i.e.: organs, tissues, glands, etc) is animated by a specific acupuncture meridian (energy channels or pathways). All the meridians run through the teeth or their sockets and in this way each tooth is related to the rest of the body by way of these energy meridians. This is slowly being accepted by mainstream doctors and dentists in the west.

As an example:

If you have a particular body part that is weak, the tooth on the same meridian could be making the problem worse or even be causing it. For instance, if you have kidney problems, a problem with tooth #3 could be making the problem worse or the kidney could be making the tooth worse. They both need to be healed eventually.

Is the unhealthy tooth or jaw bone the primary source of a physical problem or is the associated organ the cause of the bad tooth or jaw bone? Are the problems always interconnected?

Mercury In Amalgam Fillings

Mercury Toxicity Overview

The World Health Organization stated in 1990 that there is zero tolerance to mercury in the human and that the greatest source of mercury in all populations is dental amalgam.

Exposure to mercury begins in the womb where the mother transfers mercury to the fetus through the placenta. Once the fetus is out of the uterus there are many ways for mercury levels to continue accumulating as a child and adult. The common areas where mercury is found are:

Auto exhaust, Pesticides, Fertilizers, Amalgam Dental Fillings, Drinking water (tap and well), Felt, Bleached flour, Processed foods, Fabric softeners. Fish and Calomel (talc, body powder)

Mercury Fillings – How Safe Are They?

Consider these facts:

1. Mercury is the most poisonous, non-radioactive, naturally occurring substance on our planet.

2. There is *no safe or harmless level* of mercury. Just one atom of mercury is harmful to our bodies.

3. Mercury fillings continuously release poisonous mercury vapor.

4. Mercury fillings are the single greatest source of mercury exposure.

5. The first exposure to mercury from amalgam fillings can occur at the moment of conception.

6. Mercury can pass through the placenta to the fetus and through breast milk to nursing babies.

There has been much controversy over the years as to the safety of mercury fillings and most dental professionals have assumed their position on their safety based on the American Dental Association's position which I will discuss shortly.

The good news is; many dentists no longer place mercury fillings, relying instead on a number of "white-filling" alternatives because they are a better choice aesthetically and functionally nowadays. What is of concern, however, is how mercury fillings that people still have in their mouth react to their surrounding environment and if they need to be replaced.

Most people would agree that a material that has the kinds of side effects mentioned above should at the very least be studied and monitored, especially when so many people are walking around with an abundance of it in their mouths.

So, just what is the American Dental Association's stand on mercury in the mouth? Following is an excerpt taken directly from their website:

> Used by dentists for more than a century, dental amalgam is the most thoroughly researched and tested restorative material among all those in use. It is durable, easy to use, highly resistant to wear and relatively inexpensive in comparison to other materials. For those reasons, it remains a valued treatment option for dentists and their patients.
>
> Dental amalgam is a stable alloy made by combining elemental mercury, silver, tin, copper and possibly other metallic elements. Although dental amalgam continues to be a safe, commonly used restorative material, some concern has been raised because of its mercury content. However, the mercury in amalgam combines with other metals to render it stable and safe for use in filling teeth.
>
> While questions have arisen about the safety of dental amalgam relating to its mercury content, the major U.S. and international scientific and health bodies, including the National Institutes of Health, the U.S. Public Health Service, the Centers for Disease Control and Prevention, the Food and Drug Administration and the World Health Organization, among others have been satisfied that dental amalgam is a safe, reliable and effective restorative material.

History Of Mercury Amalgam

The most common dental filling materials prior to Amalgam (mercury) were: cork, tin, wood chips, resins (e.g. pine) and lead.

The word *amalgam* actually refers to any mixture of elemental mercury and other metals to form a unique compound.

Typically a compound is named after its main ingredient. In this case, the names silver or amalgam fillings were adopted. *Mercury fillings* should have been the name, as elemental mercury is the main ingredient.

1816: The first mercury filling was created by a Frenchman named August Taveau when he mixed elemental mercury with shavings from silver coins.

1830: Two French brothers, the Crawcours brought mercury fillings to England.

1833: The Crawcours emigrated to the United States bringing their mercury fillings with them.

The term dentist comes from the French word for tooth, *dent*.

Amalgam became the filling material of choice as it was *inexpensive*, easy to mix and place, sealed the tooth better and lasted longer.

Prior to 1840 there were two types of dentists: *barber-dentists* and *doctor-dentists.*

Barber-dentists probably due to their adjustable chairs were in the business of cutting hair and pulling teeth.

No training, regulations or consumer protections laws existed, and because mixing and placing mercury fillings was easy, *barber-dentists* adopted this new technique creating *healthy profits* in the process.

Doctor-dentists or physician-dentists and the rest of the scientific community of that day knew that mercury was a poison as a result of having observed chronic mercury poisoning in the hat-making industry.

Mad Hatters as they were known, were hat makers who after years of exposure to elemental mercury (a common solution used to turn fur into felt for hats contained elemental mercury) would experience mercury-related neurological symptoms such as:

>Tremors.
>Anxiety
>Emotional instability
>Mood swings and irritability
>Forgetfulness
>Insomnia
>Regressive behavior
>Aggressiveness
>Anger

Banning Elemental Mercury In Amalgam Fillings and How The American Dental Association Was Formed

Doctor-dentists had only a partial understanding of how and why elemental mercury could cause these symptoms **but** recognized at the very least that elemental mercury was a health hazard and because it was contained in amalgam fillings it should be banned!

They reasoned that if mercury could make hatters mad then what could it do to people who had it in their teeth? In an attempt to prevent unregulated barber dentists from exposing the public to this poison, doctor-dentists formed the first dental school in the U.S. in 1828 and subsequently in 1848 the first dental association, the American Society of Dental Surgeons (ASDS). In was an attempt to regulate and standardize dental treatment and give credibility to licensed dentists and here's the kicker, prohibit the use of amalgam fillings by member dentists.

A resolution was passed in 1843 banning the use of amalgam by members of the ASDS with the threat of license loss should they use amalgam. At the same time the public were still visiting barber dentists who continued to place amalgam fillings. Unfazed by the health hazards of amalgam fillings and making a great deal of money, barber-dentists were oblivious to the concerns of the ASDS.

Members of the ASDS watched as members of the public continued to visit barber-dentists to have the cheaper, longer lasting amalgam fillings placed and as a result many ASDS dentists in an attempt to cash in on the trend decided that they wanted to place amalgam fillings as well.

More and more dentists left the society in order to be able to place the highly-profitable amalgam fillings and as a result the ASDS disbanded. Then, in 1859, in what to me is a tragic and ironic twist to this story the American Dental Association (ADA) was formed to support these amalgam-placing dentists without fear of losing their licenses.

So…….. In a nutshell: Originally, based on science and health concerns, doctor-dentists tried to protect the public from mercury exposure. Now, based upon ADA statements taken directly from their website today:

> Used by dentists for more than a century, dental amalgam is the most thoroughly researched and tested restorative material among all those in use. It is durable, easy to use, highly resistant to wear and relatively inexpensive in comparison to other materials. For those reasons, it remains a valued treatment option for dentists and their patients.

Why Eliminate The Use Of Amalgam (mercury) Fillings?

My question to all of you is: Why did dentists who vehemently opposed mercury/amalgam fillings switch to their use?

From my viewpoint, it is pretty obvious that there were financial reasons. Losing money and patients to barber-dentists was the impetus to turn a blind-eye to the serious and known health hazards related to mercury fillings.

Mercury amalgam was and still is; durable, easy to use, highly resistant to wear and relatively inexpensive in comparison to other materials.

But, is it safe? History teaches us that the some early dentists still thought amalgam was unsafe and subsequently there occurred in 1926 a "Second "Amalgam War" after a German Physician, Dr. Albert Stock, showed that mercury escaped from fillings in the form of a dangerous vapor and could cause significant health issues. Again, the ADA vigorously defended the use of mercury amalgams, despite science to the contrary.

In 1986, which is now deemed the "Third Amalgam War" after pressure from mounting clinical evidence, the ADA was forced to acknowledge that mercury vapor does indeed escape from mercury fillings in patients' mouths. The ADA still insisted that mercury in those patients' mouths is safe.

However, more recent scientific studies, most of which were done in the 1990's have now revealed that:

1. Mercury in fillings continuously vaporizes into mouth air.

2. This mercury vapor is inhaled and swallowed into the body,

3. This mercury vapor is then widely distributed throughout the body, where it stays for very long periods.

4. Autopsy studies reveal a correlation between the amount of mercury in brain tissues and the number, size and number of surfaces of amalgam fillings in the mouth.

5. That mercury absorbed from these surfaces can cause changes in body chemistry and in organ functioning.

So………Where does this leave you, the public!!!! What and who do you believe?

As a member of the public you have a right to know the danger of having mercury fillings in your mouth and that today, many physicians and dentists believe that heavy metal toxicity may well be the most overlooked problem in medicine and dentistry.

Low-level exposure may simply present over the years with a *feeling* of lethargy, mild chronic headaches, possible progression into arthritis, migraines or colitis and even into debilitating diseases such as Multiple Sclerosis.

If you stand back and get some perspective on all of this, you may well see that dental personnel, working in a typical dental office, may very well be practicing in a very highly toxic and dangerous environment because of the constant, low levels of mercury they are exposed to on a daily basis.

I urge you if you have chronic health problems and still have mercury fillings in your mouth that there may be a connection. You need to find a team of health care professionals that support your health from this whole-body approach and who are willing to help you.

Should You Consider Having Your Mercury Amalgam Fillings Removed?

What is the possibility of elemental mercury exposure being an underlying component to a myriad of chronic health problems. If you were to ask most dental professionals what they think about this possibility, they would likely disagree and defer to the American Dental Association's stand on this issue; mercury/amalgam fillings are safe.

The problem may be rooted (pun intended) in the fact that the mercury exposure typically associated with amalgam fillings is a low level mercury poisoning (micromercurialism) which may present itself as: moodiness, memory loss, inability to concentrate, anxiety and even severe depression, all symptoms that are commonly thought to be caused by stress or aging. But, some believe otherwise!

> "Chronic, low-level heavy metal poisoning, especially with mercury, is a major health problem that has been virtually unrecognized. As I have been testing for mercury poisoning, I am seeing heavy metal toxicity with increasing frequency, especially in patients with chronic degenerative diseases, chronic fatigue, fibromyalgia, allergies, hypertension and autoimmune disease. It is crucial to well-being to recognize this health threat." Robban Sica M.D.

I would also like to touch briefly on another threat related to mercury/amalgam fillings which has to do with its electrical conductivity. It is a known scientific fact that when you place two different metals in a salt solution, similar to saliva, an electrical charge is created and essentially a battery has formed in the mouth. This phenomenon has been recognized for many years and is referred to as Galvanic Current or Galvanism. Mercury amalgam is typically made of five metals which are of concern on its own, but, add a gold or silver crown in the mouth and the electricity generated may increase/alter significantly.

We are energetic beings and at every minute billions of electrical impulses are messaging through our body, organizing and supporting a series of highly-complex bodily processes. It is logical to reason that any electrical interference coming from our mouth might be creating disharmony and interfering with normal electrical signals.

Following is a list of symptoms caused by Galvanic Current taken directly from a study by E.S. Lain, et al, and published in the Journal of the American Dental Association (JADA) in 1936:

1. Metallic or salty taste.

2. Increased saliva.

3. Burning or tingling sensation along the tongue.

4. Occasional nerve shocks and pulp sensitivity from connecting restorations or by connections made with a spoon or fork.

5. Pathological changes in blood, kidney or organs, probably caused by absorption of ionized toxic metals.

6. Generalized discomfort in the mouth, irritability, indigestion, loss of weight and in some cases, reflex radiating neurologic pains through branches of the fifth cranial nerve (trigeminal nerve).

So…… if you are experiencing any of these symptoms and *feel* that they may be related to conditions in your mouth, I suggest you begin by speaking to your dental professional about your concerns and consider finding a Holistic Dentist.

Removing Mercury Amalgam Fillings; Mercury Toxicity And Chronic Health Issues

Many people may decide to have their mercury amalgams removed for preventive reasons. There are also a good many people who may be experiencing chronic health issues that are related to heavy metal toxicity.

I have recently read "The Swiss Secret to Optimal Health" by Thomas Rau M.D.. Lauded as the "Mozart of medicine", Dr. Rau is the world's foremost practitioner of biological medicine. He is the medical director of the Paracelsus Clinic in Switzerland and his program has proven effective time and again, especially for those with chronic conditions like allergies, arthritis, heart disease, high blood pressure, diabetes and even cancer.

Swiss biological medicine is holistic in that it sees each individual as unique and as a complete entity. To effect a permanent solution, the symptom experienced by the patient needs an interpreter to divine its origin. Swiss biological medicine strives to diagnose and remove the underlying *cause* or *causes,* of an ailment.

Dr. Rau points out in his book that, "Very often, we find hidden causes for chronic diseases in the teeth. Heavy metals from amalgam fillings and toxins from subclinical infections from old root canals are frequent causes of symptoms and impediments to healing. Even trace amounts of mercury in the system for example, can lead to colitis, sinusitis or asthma".

No matter how you have come to the decision, I urge you to choose who will remove your fillings and how, very carefully. What you want to look for is a mercury safe dentist and since a universal consensus on protocol has yet to be reached for minimizing a patient's exposure to mercury during removal, this could be a little difficult.

Remember, no dentist is under any legal obligation to provide patients with protection against mercury exposure during the removal process. Mercury safe dentists provide different levels of protection to their clients because they believe it is the ethically right thing to do. They believe these fillings are a health hazard to the client, the office staff where they are being removed as well as the environment.

Adapted by author from (Kathleen Bernardi. <http://woodlanddental.ca/press/>
See six separate web pages in references

Holistic Vs. Conventional Dentistry

There is no difference between a holistic or biological dentist and a conventional or traditional one in terms of basic training. Both have fulfilled comparable educational and licensing requirements. Both have demonstrated an understanding of dentistry as it has been taught , practiced and approved by the American Dental Association., They get their license when they have demonstrated skill level sufficient to earn the title of DDS (Doctor of Dental Surgery) or DMD (Dental Medical Doctor).

Most holistic dentists began their careers practicing in the traditional manner and later incorporated holistic procedures as their awareness grew regarding the nature, effectiveness and dangers of current conventional dentistry as approved by the American Dental Association. This new awareness could have been facilitated by a seminar on holistic dentistry or first-hand experience of the toxic effects of mercury and other common dental practices.

The holistic dentist has dared to step outside the traditional dental paradigm and look at the whole-body effect of routine dental procedures. S/he is far more than a "tooth mechanic." S/he is a doctor in the truest sense, one who is guided by the cardinal rule of the Hippocratic oath, "First, do no harm."

CONVENTIONAL (ADA) DENTAL PRACTICES	HOLISTIC OR BIOLOGICAL DENTAL PRACTICES
Uses "silver" amalgams, which are half mercury. Denies the health risks of using such fillings. ADA claim: Replacement of amalgams is "unethical."	**Never uses amalgam** fillings; will replace amalgams for health reasons (using precautions) if the patient wants it done. Is aware of the adverse health impact of amalgams and seeks to understand the health impact of all dental work on the body and the brain.
Nickel (a component of stainless steel is routinely used in dentures and braces. Gold fillings and crowns may be placed into the mouth along with amalgams, creating a "battery effect" from the currents generated by dissimilar metals. All materials are used without regard to toxicity, allergy or biocompatibility.	**Nickel is avoided** in crowns and other dental applications because it is a neurotoxin (poison to the nervous system) and carcinogen (cancer-causing substance). **Gold alloys are either avoided or used only after compatibility testing,** as gold is a conducting metal and always contains other metals, some toxic. Gold is never used when amalgams are present in the mouth.
May be improperly trained on how to properly place composite (tooth-colored) filling material, increasing the failure rate.	Relies on ceramics for inlays, onlays and crowns and uses carefully selected composites for direct fillings.
Is likely unfamiliar with biocompatibility testing. Therefore may deny that biocompatibility of materials used is important to health.	**Uses biocompatibility testing** routinely to determine what filling, crown or bridge materials are most compatible with patient's unique body chemistry (and thus will be least likely to trigger an immune response).
Typically uses inadequate precautions or no precautions when replacing old amalgam fillings.	**Takes elaborate precautions when drilling out old amalgam fillings.**
Usually unaware of the health risks associated with standard dental materials and procedures. May scoff at health concerns when raised; has dangerous levels of mercury vapor in the dental clinic. The dentist, hygienist and assistant may all have high mercury levels in their bodies, adversely affecting their health.	Collaborates with naturopathic physicians or holistic medical doctors to help evaluate the health status of the patient and to plot a strategy for safe dental work and for detoxification. **Encourages baseline testing and evaluation for heavy metal toxicity**; recognizes possible need for medical preparation before amalgams are replaced.

CONVENTIONAL (ADA) DENTAL PRACTICES	HOLISTIC OR BIOLOGICAL DENTAL PRACTICES
Does root canal treatments, typically using gutta percha as a filling material for root canals; denies any health hazards associated with root canal treatment.	Many **avoid the risks of root canal** fillings by extracting the dead tooth and putting in a bridge or partial denture. Some use alternative filling materials in the root canal.
When extracting a tooth, will most likely leave a portion of the bony socket and a portion of periodontal ligament, which connects tooth to bone.	After tooth extraction, takes care to **thoroughly remove the periodontal ligament** by scraping the bony socket down to healthy bone to prevent jawbone infection and promote healing.
Is unfamiliar with jawbone "cavitations," or downplays their prevalence and is therefore apt to miss their presence, even when indicators and risk factors are present.	**Recognizes that jawbone cavitations frequently occur** where teeth have been extracted, where there have been root canal treated teeth and where other risk factors are present. Either scans for cavitations him/herself or refers to others equipped to do so and to perform surgery or other appropriate treatment.
Recognizes periodontal disease as a threat to teeth and to general health. Likely to use surgery or "root planing" as a primary treatment.	Recognizes periodontal disease as a threat to teeth and to general health. Typically uses herbal and other rinses to treat the infection, **but avoids antibiotic use, surgery and root planning**. Avoids using surgery to remove potentially healthy gum tissue.
Advocates the use of fluoridated toothpastes, gels, mouthwashes and fluoridated water. The American Dental Association receives millions in revenue for placing its "Seal of Acceptance" on fluoridated products.	Avoids use of fluoridated dental products, as fluoride is toxic and accumulates in the body. Recognizes dental fluorosis (discoloration of children's teeth) as a sign of systemic fluoride poisoning. Opposes water fluoridation due to documented health hazards.

Adapted by author from <http://healthcarealternatives.net/conholistic.html > in about 2001. The website is no longer active as of November 2013.

Tooth To Organs And Emotions Chart

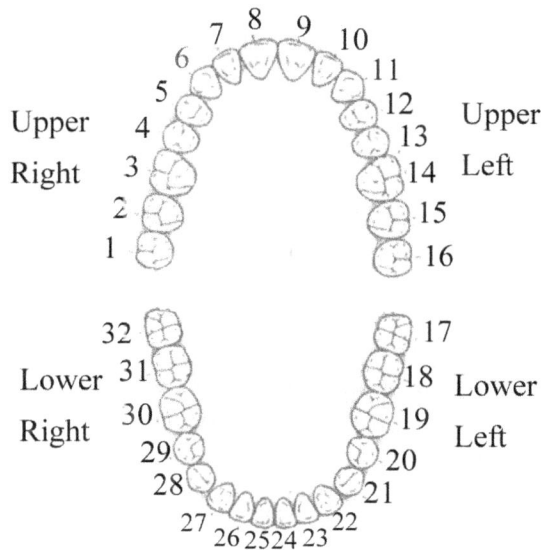

The author created this table from Oasis Advanced Wellness. 17 December 2013 and Thieves oil blend - Arm yourself with the power of Thieves 17 December 2013

To use this chart look up the tooth that is bothering you from the picture above. Then find it in the left column below.

Tooth	Meridian	Organs & Glands	Positive Emotions	Negative Emotions
1 -Third Molar (top right Wisdom Tooth)	small intestine	Duodenum Heart pituitary anterior lobe	Love Joy Compassion	Resentment Rejection Family Problems
2 -Second Molar (top right)	stomach	adrenal Bladder Pancreas parathyroid pineal Stomach	Security Self-Esteem Order	Guilt Low Self-Esteem Judgmental Depression

Tooth	Meridian	Organs & Glands	Positive Emotions	Negative Emotions
3 - First Molar (top right)	stomach	Kidneys Liver Pancreas pituitary Stomach thyroid	Resolution Determination Caring Humor	Unflexibility Anger Pride Disrespectful
4 - Second Premolar (top right)	large intestine	Duodenum Gall Bladder Intestine - Large Intestine - Small Lung - Right thymus thyroid	Ego Determination Balance Passion	Critical Possessiveness Revenge Monotony
5 - First Premolar (top right)	large intestine	Intestine - Large Lung - Right Pancreas pituitary posterior lobe Stomach thyroid	Self-Esteem Excitement Purpose Affection	Unacceptance Grief Condemnation Pain Love
6 - Canine (top right)	gall bladder/liver	Gall Bladder Heart Liver pituitary posterior lobe	Joy Compassion Decisiveness Pride	Family Problems Regret Anger Rejection
7 - Second Incisor (top right)	bladder	Bladder Kidney - Right pineal Urogenital	Intimacy Caring Order	Ego Problems Inflexibility Aloof Disorganized
8 - First Incisor (top right)	bladder/kidney	Bladder epididymis Kidney - Right pineal Urogenital	Acceptance Clarity Survival	Emotional Outbursts Disrespect Stubbornness

Tooth	Meridian	Organs & Glands	Positive Emotions	Negative Emotions
9 - First Incisor (top left)	bladder/ kidney	Bladder epididymis Kidney - Left pineal Urogenital	Intimacy Acceptance Order	Ego Problems Inflexibility Survival Fear
10 - Second Incisor (top left)	bladder	Bladder Kidney - Left pineal Urogenital	Survival Comforting Closeness	Stuborness Prideful Avoidance of Intimacy Repression
11 - Canine (top left)	gall bladder/ liver	Bile Ducts Heart Liver pituitary posterior lobe	Love Purpose Resolution Approval	Sadness Regret Anger Critical Resentment
12 - First Premolar (top left)	large intestine	Intestine - Large Liver Lung - Left Pancreas pituitary posterior lobe Stomach thyroid	Happiness Decisiveness Excitement Judgment	Depression Controlling Grief Monotony Spite
13 - Second Premolar (top left)	large intestine	Duodenum Gall Bladder Intestine - Large Intestine - Small Liver Lung - Left thymus thyroid	Balance Assimilation Determination Enthusiasm	Anti-social Fear Uneasiness Negativity Unacceptance

Tooth	Meridian	Organs & Glands	Positive Emotions	Negative Emotions
14 - First Molar (top left)	stomach	Kidneys Liver pituitary Stomach thyroid	Comforting Purpose Affection Peace	Regret Self-Condemenation Agitation Rejection Price
15 - Second Molar (top left)	stomach	adrenal Bladder parathyroid pineal Spleen Stomach	Security Closeness Self-Love Calmness	Lack of Self-love Antagonism Emotional Conflict
16 - Third Molar (top left Wisdom Tooth)	small intestine	Heart Ileum Jejunum pituitary anterior lobe	Compassion Love Joy	Avoidance Rejection Resentment
17 - Third Molar (bottom left Wisdom Tooth)	small intestine	Heart Jejunum Liver	Joy Resolution Love Purpose	Depression Guilt Family Problems Regret
18 - Second Molar (bottom left)	large intestine	appendages Bladder Pancreas pineal Stomach	Assimilation Passion Excitement	Manipulative Anger Self-centered Grief
19 - First Molar (bottom left)	large intestine	Intestine - Large Lungs pituitary	Balance Enthusiasm Zest	Controlling Love Pain Over Critical Revenge
20 - Second Premolar (bottom left)	stomach	Spleen Stomach thyroid	Calmness Peace Happiness	Agitation Condemnation Unrestful Emotional Conflicts

Tooth	Meridian	Organs & Glands	Positive Emotions	Negative Emotions
21 - First Premolar (bottom left)	stomach	Gonads Liver Pancreas Spleen Stomach	Enthusiasm Humor Self Love Security	Lack of Self-love Resentment Anger Regret
22 - Canine (bottom left)	gall bladder/ liver	Bile Ducts Gonads Liver Lungs Pancreas	Resolution Excitment Judgment	Over-bearing Resentment Disorganized Lack of Acceptance
23 - Second Incisor (bottom left)	bladder	adrenals Bladder Kidney - Left Urogenital	Order Closeness Comforting Caring	Pride Repression Unhappy Sexual *Feelings*
24 - First Incisor (bottom left)	bladder	adrenals Bladder epididymis Kidney - Left Urogenital	Intimacy Acceptance Order	Anger Inflexibility Emotional Outbursts
25 - First Incisor (bottom right)	bladder/ kidney	adrenals Bladder epididymis Kidney - Right Urogenital	Acceptance Clarity Survival	Stubbornness Disrespect Sexual Problems
26 - Second Incisor (bottom right)	bladder	adrenals Bladder Kidney - Right Urogenital	Intimacy Caring Order	Inflexible Disorganized Disharmony
27 - Canine (bottom right)	gall bladder/ liver	Gall Bladder gonads Liver Lungs Pancreas	Joy Pride Judgment Decisiveness Compassion	Condemnation Family Problems Anger Regret Grief

Tooth	Meridian	Organs & Glands	Positive Emotions	Negative Emotions
28 - First Premolar (bottom right)	stomach	gonads Liver Pancreas Pylorus Stomach	Self-Esteem Purpose Affection	Insecurity Low Self-esteem Judgmental, Regret Pushy
29 - Second Premolar (bottom right)	stomach	Duodenum Gall Bladder Intestine - Large Intestine - Small Liver Lung - Right thyroid	Balance Ego Determination Passion	Unyielding Unforgiving Manipulative Revenge Controlling
30 - First Molar (bottom right)	large intestine	Ileocecal Region Intestine - Large pituitary	Balance Passion Zest	Pessimistic Anti-social Fear of the Future Grief
31 - Second Molar (bottom right)	large intestine	appendages Ileocecal Region Intestine - Large Lungs pineal	Passion Balance Excitement	Negativity Lack of Acceptance Guilt Deppression
32 - Third Molar (bottom right Wisdom Tooth)	small intestine	Heart Ileocecal Region Ileum	Joy Compassion Love Approval	Family Problems Avoidance Resentment

Created by the author from information found on the internet at

<http://www.oasisadvancedwellness.com/tools/tooth-chart-top.htm#01> 17 December 2013

<http://www.oasisadvancedwellness.com/tools/tooth-chart-btm.htm#17> 17 December 2013

<http://www.secretofthieves.com/tooth-chart/index.cfm> 17 December 2013

Cavitations

What Are Cavitations? How Common Are They? What Are Their Chronic Health Effects?

A cavitation is a hole in the bone, often where a tooth has been removed and the bone has a dead, hollow, area. In the last several years, the term cavitation has been used to describe various bone lesions which appear both as empty holes in the jawbones and holes filled with dead bone and bone marrow. Dead, cavitational areas, which produce pain, are now called NICO (Neuralgia Inducing Osteonecrosis) lesions.

When a tooth is being extracted, in what has been normal dental procedure, the surrounding periodontal membrane is usually left behind. Theoretically, when a tooth has been pulled, the body will eventually fill in the space in the bone where the tooth once was. **But** when the membrane is left behind, an incomplete healing commonly takes place which leaves a hole or a spongy place inside the jaw bone. Experts speculate that perhaps this is because the bone cells on either side sense the presence of the periodontal membrane and "think" that the tooth is still there. This appears to be one common cause of cavitations.

A cavitation can form in any bone in the body. There are also other reasons that cavitations form, some of which are localized traumas, poor circulation to the area, clotting disorders, and the use of steroids.

What's Hiding Inside?

Inside a cavitation, bacteria flourish and deviant cells multiply. Cavitations act as a breeding ground for bacteria and their toxins. Research has shown these bacterial waste products to be extremely potent. Cavitations can also cause blockages on the body's energy meridians and can exert far-reaching impacts on the overall system. Investigation has revealed that some cavitations are reservoirs of huge amounts of mercury and other toxic substances. Cavitations may be a source of low level or high level stress on the entire body.

How Toxic Are Cavitations And What Type Of Effects Are Caused By Cavitations?

There are indications that other types of toxins also accumulate in cavitations, and when these toxins combine with certain chemicals or heavy metals (for example, mercury), much more potent toxins may form.

High levels of mercury are commonly found in some cavitations and in general in the jawbone of those with mercury amalgam fillings and to have significant local and systemic effects. Mercury is known to be extremely toxic and to commonly cause chronic adverse local and systemic health effects. Yeast and fungi have also been found to accumulate in cavitations, and to have significant systemic effects.

Cavitations Are Very Common

Bob Jones is the inventor of the Cavitat - an ultrasound instrument designed to detect and image cavitations that has been approved for testing for cavitations by the FDA after undergoing FDA clinical trials. He found cavitations of various sizes and severity in approximately 94% of several thousand wisdom teeth sites scanned. He also found cavitations under or located near over 90% of root canal teeth scanned in both males and females of various ages from several different geographic areas of the United States. Note again that the population being tested for cavitations in these trials is different than the general population, which might have a somewhat lower incidence of cavitations. **But** it's clear that the occurrence is very common. (Glenn's note: I met Bob Jones when he was showing my dentist, who is now retired, how to use the Cavitat. It found two cavitations that were impossible to see on X-Rays or MRIs. As of 2013 there are only about twelve Cavitat machines in use in the United States because of harassment from the American Dental Association.)

Root Canals And Cavitations

Research has demonstrated that virtually all root canals result in residual infection due to the imperfect seal that allows bacteria to penetrate.

The toxins given off by these bacteria are often even more toxic than mercury. The bacterial toxins from root-canalled teeth and associated cavitations can cause systemic diseases of the heart, kidney and uterus as well as to the immune, nervous and endocrine systems.

Biopsies of bone material collected from cavitation surgeries have most often shown osteonecrosis, or dead bone material.

Many researchers today believe that NICO lesions, like periodontal disease, is the focus of various infections which may spread throughout the body and have systemic effects. In the last few years, some of the most surprising medical news has been the discovery that bacteria from the mouth appear to be very influential in causing various heart, liver, kidney, and immune problems.

From <http://www.flcv.com/cavitati.html> December 2013

Nutrition

The Basics

There is a general consensus that eating too many cookies, cakes and sweets is unhealthy. Almost everything else has controversy to some extent.

The controversy about 'living water' and 'dead water is in heated debate as well as the heated debate about GMO (Genetically Modified) foods.. What I present here are my conclusions and beliefs.

I got the information from many sources and put much of it together for myself before I realized I would be writing this.

Most of the Nutrition information without sources cited was gathered by studying *The Blood Type Diet* developed by Peter D'Adamo, *The Zone Diet* developed by Barry Sears and The Metabolic Typing Diet as explained in *The Metabolic Typing Diet* by William Wolcott and Trish Fahey and developed as follows. In the 1930's, dentist Weston Price began expeditions around the world and uncovered the link between modern eating habits and chronic degenerative diseases. He also discovered that there was no one diet that would be healthy for all people -- there was too much variation in climate, local produce, environmental conditions, heredity, genetics and culture. In later years, George Watson, Roger Williams, William Kelley, and others continued research in this area. They believed that people's metabolisms functioned differently and the differences are largely determined by heredity.

Seven Major Hidden Food Allergens:

dairy, soy, corn, eggs, chocolate (cocoa), gluten (especially wheat gluten) and peanuts.

Gluten Containing Grains:

<u>Wheat, Barley and Rye</u>: the three most common gluten intolerances.

Wheat, barley and rye are the three main gluten-containing grains. The gluten in wheat is named gliadin, while the type of gluten in barley is named hordein and the one in rye is secalin. Other species of wheat, such as triticale, kamut and spelt, also contain gluten. All foods made from these grains or the flours made from these grains provide gluten and are unsuitable for a gluten-free diet. For example, wheat products such as couscous, bulgur, pasta, bread, pizza dough, crackers and baked goods are all examples of gluten-rich foods.

<u>Oats</u>: a type of gluten that is usually well tolerated by most people with gluten intolerance

Oats contain avenin, a type of gluten that is usually tolerated by most people with celiac disease or gluten intolerance. However, most oats that are processed in the United States are processed in the same facilities where wheat and other gluten-containing grains are treated. As a result, most oats sold in the U.S. are contaminated with wheat, barley or rye gluten. Choose certified gluten-free oats if you are following a gluten-free diet to prevent introducing gluten in your diet.

<u>Buckwheat, Quinoa and Millet</u>: All three are gluten-free and are perfect options for your gluten-free diet.

Millet is a cereal grain, which are grasses with a mildly sweet, nutty flavor. Buckwheat is a green, leafy, flowering plant. Quinoa is a relative of leafy green vegetables, like spinach and Swiss chard and Quinoa's small, plentiful seeds can be used much like cereal grains.

You can use these 'grains' to replace gluten-containing grains and you will see that some gluten-free products are made from these gluten-free 'grains'. You can make bread and baked goods with buckwheat, use millet instead of pasta to prepare a cold salad and cook quinoa to serve as a porridge for breakfast instead of gluten-contaminated oats.

<u>Rice and Corn</u> are gluten-free grains (Be aware that about 90% of corn is GMO)

Rice and corn are two gluten-free grains. Your gluten-free diet can use rice-based pasta and noodles instead of the wheat-based option. Sushi, rice and vegetable stir-fries, and chicken and rice soup are appropriate gluten-free dishes. Although corn is often consumed as a vegetable, it actually is a grain and can be part of your gluten-free diet, whether you have it on the cob, creamed or popped. You can also experiment with other gluten-free grains, such as sorghum and teff.

Eat Whole Grains Only.

Nitrites: are unhealthy, period (ham, lunch meats, bacon, and other "cured" foods)

Prunes, Apples and Pears: are very high in sorbitol which can cause diarrhea and flatulence

Artificial Sweeteners, MSG, Food Colorings and Preservatives.

It is best to avoid all artificial and man manipulated ingredients. This includes 'natural flavors', red, blue and yellow dyes, caramel coloring and high fructose corn syrup. A special note on 'natural': Natural and artificial flavors have very different names and yet are very similar. Both types of flavors are derived from chemicals in laboratories. The difference is that 'natural flavors' are a mix of natural chemicals and that artificial flavors are obtained from synthetic chemicals. Natural chemicals are still chemicals. Artificial flavoring might actually be better for you, because chemicals used in these flavorings have passed safety tests.

Do Your Best To Eliminate:

Wheat, White Sugar, Caffeine (except for Green Tea), all artificial sweeteners, alcohol, all dairy except Greek Yogurt and meals between 8 PM and 8 AM. If you are on shift work adjust times to match your sleeping schedule.

Start Your Day:

with cup hot water & ½ lemon squeezed into the water to keep the kidneys and liver clean and functioning well.

Eat A Healthy Breakfast.

Protein, Carbohydrates and Good Fats Ratios:

Protein, carbohydrates and good fats ratios vary according to the individual.

The ratio of protein to good fats should be about equal by calories (1 to 1).

Which is the same as 10 grams Protein to 4 grams good fat (1 to 0.4).

The normal range **by calories** is from:

20% protein+20%good fat+60% good carbohydrates to
40% protein+40%good fat+20% good carbohydrates.

Additional Information On Foods

Phytates (Phytic Acid)

Phytic acid in food reduces your body's ability to absorb the minerals the food has to offer. Although phytates do bind with minerals, they may actually be preventing the formation of free radicals, thereby keeping the minerals at safe levels in the body. Phytates also have a role to play in cell growth and can move excess minerals out of the body.

There are methods of preparing grains and legumes that reduce the phytic acid content and improve mineral absorption.

The soybean has one of the highest phytate levels of any grain or legume that has been studied and the phytates in soy are highly resistant to normal phytate-reducing techniques such as long, slow cooking. Only a long period of fermentation will significantly reduce the phytate content of soybeans.

Soymilk and Tofu:

Soybeans in soymilk are soaked, strained, and cooked. Tofu has an additional step ; a coagulant is added. Both of these products retain nearly 100% of the phytates.

Ferment Soy to reduce the phytic acid content. Soaking and boiling soybeans leaves the full amount of phytic acid in the bean.

Stick with Fermented Tempeh and Miso

See "Soy as an Enzyme Inhibitor" later in this chapter

Beans:

Simply cooking beans that are high in Phytates is ineffective in reducing phytate levels appreciably, as is sprouting.

Your best bet is a warm, 18-hour soak and drain prior to cooking in fresh water.

Foods With Significant Amounts Of Phytates

Vegetables and Legumes With Significant Amounts of Phytates

Soybean   (All unfermented Soy, including Tofu, Shoyu and Edamame)
Beans   (adzuki, black, mung, broad, fava, copper, tamarind, Cranberry, garbanzo, green, northern, jicama, , Lima, navy, pink, winged, Pinto, Soybean, tara, white, French, Yambean, yellow, mothbeans)
Peas   (green, pod, snow, black-eyed, cowpeas, chickpeas, Pigeon)
Carob
Lentils
Lupins

Nuts (Almonds, Cashews, Hazelnuts, peanuts, black walnuts)

Reducing phytic acid in nuts and seeds is tricky. Soaking nuts is recommended. The problem is that a nut has a small surface area. It would be better to grind the nut at least slightly before soaking it. You then have nuts pieces.

Grains With Significant Amounts of Phytates

Alfalfa (sprouted), Amaranth, Arrowroot, Artichoke, Barley, Buckwheat, Bulgur Wheat, Couscous(cracked wheat), Kamut, Kasha (dish made with buckwheat), Millet, Oats, Quinoa, Rice, Rye, Semolina, Sorghum, Spelt, Tapioca, Teff, Tritacale, Wheat

Thiocyante

If you have thyroid problems or trouble utilizing iodine you may want to limit Thiocyanate in your diet. It can worsen thyroid dysfunction and inhibits iodine metabolism.

Dietary or nutritional thiocyanate is a very important substance that is necessary for optimal health and wellbeing for Africans and people of African descent, as well as all naturally dark skinned people.

Thiocyanate is found in specific foods common to the African diet as well as some Middle Eastern and Mediterranean diets.

Thiocyanate is a must have substance if one is dealing with the challenge of sickle cell anemia.

Dietary Thiocyanate is an anti-sickling agent as well as having antibiotic activity.

Foods With Significant Amounts of Thiocyanate

Broccoli, Brussels Sprouts, Cabbage (Chinese, red, white), Cauliflower, Kale, Mustard Greens, Rutabaga, Watercress

Oxalic Acid

When you eat foods containing oxalic acid, this substance can interfere with the absorption of minerals, such as calcium, magnesium and potassium. Oxalic acid also can combine with minerals in the body, creating oxalate crystals that may cause problems for people prone to kidney or bladder stones or gout.

FoodS High In Oxalic Acid

Rhubarb

Levels of Oxalic Acid are so high in rhubarb leaves that they're poisonous even if cooked.

Fruits With Significant Amounts of Oxalic Acid

Apples, Blackberry, Cranberry, Currants (black, red), Gooseberry, Grapes (All), Raspberry, Strawberry, Plums (dark, green, red)

Sweets and Condiments With Significant Amounts of Oxalic Acid

Chocolate, Cocoa

Beverages With Significant Amounts of Oxalic Acid

Tea (black- regular and decaf)

Cooking

The oxalic acid in vegetables is broken down in cooking, which then allows absorption of calcium present in other foods that you might eat at the same time.

Purine

Plant purines are far safer than meat and fish purines in terms of gout risk.

Enjoy all of these foods, with an emphasis on healthy choices unless you are at risk for gout or health problems related to purine-related metabolism. In general, we want purines in our diet. Our bodies can break purines down into uric acid, a substance that can help protect our blood vessels from damage.

If you need to follow a strict, low-purine diet because of gouty arthritis, you'll want to limit your consumption of animal foods, fish, and lentils. There are rare conditions in which metabolism of purines in the body gets disrupted. These problems include, especially in children, anemia, failure to thrive, autism, cerebral palsy, deafness, epilepsy, susceptibility to recurrent infection, and the inability to walk or talk.

Cooking To Reduce Purine Content

Boiling or steaming high-purine foods in water can cause break-down of the purine-containing components and reduces the purine risk. Baking or broiling is far less effective.

Foods With Very High Purine Content

Meats With Very High Purine Content

Brain (Organ), Buffalo, Heart (Organ), Kidney (Organ), Liver (Organ), Squirrel, Sweetbreads (various organ meats), Venison

Poultry With Very High Purine Content

Goose, Ostrich, Partridge, Pheasant, Squab (Pigeon)

Seafood With Very High Purine Content

Herring, Mussels, Sardine, Smelt

Other Foods With Very High Purine Content

Fat (beef tallow, chicken, duck, goose, lard, mutton tallow, turkey), Yeast (bakers, brewers)

Meats With High Purine Content

Bacon and Canadian Bacon, Beef, Goat, Ham (any kind), Lamb, Mutton, Pork (any), Rabbit, Sheep, Tripe (Stomach), Veal

Poultry With High Purine Content

Chicken (dark Meat), Cornish hens, Duck, Guinea Hen, Quail, Turkey (white and dark meat)

Seafood With High Purine Content

Anchovy, Bass (Sea, Striped, Small Mouth, Large Mouth), Beluga, Bluefish, Bluegill bass, Bullhead, Burbot, Butterfish, Carp, Catfish, Caviar, Chub, Cisco, Cod, Crab, Croaker, Cusk, Cutlefish, Dolphin (Mahi-Mahi), Drum, Flounder, Gray sole, Grouper, Haddock, Hake, Halfmoon, Halibut, Harvest Fish, Ling, Lobster, Mackerel, Mahi-mahi, Milkfish, Mullet, Ocean Pout, Opaleye, Orange Roughy, Oysters, Parrotfish, Perch, Perch (Ocean, White, Yellow, Silver), Pickerel, Pike, Pompano, Porgy, Red Snapper, Rosefish, Sablefish, Sailfish, Salmon, Scallop, Scrod, Scup, Shark, Sheepshead, Shrimp, Snail, Snapper, Sole, Spiny Lobster, Spot, Squid (calamari), Sturgeon, Sucker, Sunfish, Surimi, Swordfish, Tilapia, Tilefish, Trout (Rainbow, Sea, Brook), Tuna, Turbot, Weakfish, Whelk, Whitefish, Whiting, Wolffish, Yellowtail

Vegetables and Legumes With High Purine Content

Asparagus, Beans (Kidney, Lima, Navy), Cauliflower, Lentils (all), Mushrooms, Peas, Spinach

Grains With High Purine Content

Oatmeal

Soy As An Enzyme Inhibitor

Soybean in any form that is improperly fermented or unfermented including Soy Protein Isolate, Tofu, Tamari, Edamame and Shoyu acts as an enzyme inhibitor and is best avoided.

Fermentation Releases Nutrients And Transforms Soybeans Into Nutritious Food

The first soy foods were fermented products like tempeh, natto, miso and soy sauce sometime during the Chou Dynasty. Until then it was avoided as a food.

Soy also has one of the highest phytate levels of any grain or legume that has been studied (see Phytates above)

The Chinese avoided eating unfermented soybeans because the soybean contains large quantities of natural toxins or "anti-nutrients". First among them are potent enzyme inhibitors that block the action of trypsin and other enzymes needed for protein digestion.

These inhibitors can produce serious gastric distress, reduced protein digestion and chronic deficiencies in amino acid uptake.

Vegetarians who consume tofu and bean curd as a substitute for meat and dairy products risk severe mineral deficiencies. These include calcium, magnesium, iron and especially zinc.

Zinc is called the intelligence mineral because it is needed for optimal development and functioning of the brain and nervous system. It plays a role in protein synthesis and collagen formation; it is involved in the blood-sugar control mechanism and thus protects against diabetes; it is needed for a healthy reproductive system. Zinc is a key component in numerous vital enzymes and plays a role in the immune system.

Phytoestrogens In Soy

Soy milk, tofu, vegetarian meat and cheese substitutes made with soy, soy flour and soy supplements in the form of capsules or powders all supply phytoestrogens.

Soy's phytoestrogens provide adverse effects on various human tissues. High levels of phytoestrogen impair fertility. For men, it decreases the amount of testosterone, thus affecting sperm production.

Phytoestrogen mimics the effects of the female hormone estrogen. And this alters a woman's menstrual cycle as well as disrupts endocrine functionality, which can promote infertility and breast cancer. Children become highly susceptible to early maturation (which leads to early puberty) due to these hormones, and more growth and reproductive problems can happen when they reach puberty.

Other health risks of drinking soy milk may include development of kidney stones, weakening of the immune system, developing soy allergens and digestive intolerance. The anti-nutrients due to the phytic acid content of soy can also lead to osteoporosis later in life.

Other Things Some People May Want To Be Aware Of:

Glycemic index (important to stabilize blood sugar)

Volumetrics (some things are more filling with fewer calories)

Water

Water is one of the most important factors for your health, especially when you consider that your body actually consists of over 99 percent water molecules. I believe water is a really underappreciated part of the equation of Nutrition and optimal health.

Living Water

One of the key ingredients to create living water is *light (* electromagnetic energy, whether in the form of visible light, ultraviolet (UV) wavelengths and infrared wavelengths) which we're surrounded by all the time.

Living water is alkaline and carries a negative charge. Maintaining this state of alkalinity and negative charge appears to be important for optimal health. Drinking water can be optimized in a variety of different ways.

Natural spring water is an excellent way to obtain healthy water.

<http:/FindaSpring.com> can help you find a natural spring close to you.

Spring water when you drink it right out of the spring may be healthy 'dead water'. To be considered 'living water', it must either run along for sometime on the surface or first be kept for three hours or so in a wooden or clay vessel with a wide neck. Living water needs to absorb sunlight. With the aid of sunlight, microbes and bacteria are generated which are indispensable to human life. Then the water should stand in the shade for at least another three hours. After that it can be drunk as 'living water'.

Natural living water is surface water from pure streams or bodies of water, a few of which have been preserved.

Living water is clean and pure, full of energy, infused with oxygen, rich with minerals and Ph balanced to match your body fluids.

'Dead Water' can be brought very close to 'Living Water' by adding a small amount of natural sea salt that has never been heated. The salt can be recognized by its off white color and visible specks of minerals. You can also buy drops to add to the water. There are different alkalizing and mineralizing drops and supplements you can had to water. One of the best is made for BioProtien Technology of Tempe, Florida and called "Hydro Cell" <http://www.bioproteintech.com>. Something very similar (H²O Alive™) is available at Good Health Supplement in Sedona, Arizona <http://www.goodhealthsupplements.com>.

In addition to avoiding tap water with chemicals, one must also be careful of softened, distilled, reverse osmosis or other overly filtered water. These systems remove too many of the minerals. In turn, this water will leach minerals from your body and possibly leave you in a depleted condition. If you drink (or cook with) water softened with salt it is like a big salt shaker. Drinking living water hydrates cells and improves health. Drinking overly filtered water can actually dehydrate cells.

You can also help generate an electron surplus and support this negative charge within your body, by simply connecting to the Earth, which *also* has a negative charge. This is the basis of grounding techniques, which have significant health benefits. It's as though your cells are built like batteries that are naturally recharged by spending time outdoors and walking barefoot, connecting to the negative charge of the earth! This allows the transfer of negatively charged electrons from the ground into the soles of your feet.

If you have an organ that's functioning poorly, the negative charge from the earth and drinking living water can help restore the negative charge and assist the organ in healing.

Dead Water

Sometimes you need to drink dead water (avoid if polluted) because it contains very few microbes. It will rinse your insides and cleanse them, washing out a lot of microbes and bacteria from your body Then drink living water and all the microbes and bacteria you need will be restored in a balance that is just right for you.

Adapted by author from <http://articles.mercola.com/sites/articles/archive/2013/08/18/exclusion-zone-water.aspx> and Vladimir Megre, Book # 8.1: *The New Civilization,* pages 40 and 41 of The Ringing Cedars Series

Heirloom Seeds

Please note that store-bought seeds available in America and elsewhere in the 'civilized world' are often coated with a poison or toxic substance for ease of storage, and should never be used if you are doing your best to be as natural as possible. They also often come from hybrid or even GMO stock. If you wish to follow best planting advice, be sure to use your own seeds or procure *organic* seeds from a reputable producer. Heirloom organic seeds are the healthiest and if they are from a local source they will be the most hearty in the area.

Before the industrialization of agriculture, a much wider variety of plant foods were grown for human consumption. In modern agriculture in the industrialized world, most food crops are now grown in large, monocultural plots. In order to maximize consistency, few varieties of each type of crop are grown. These varieties are often selected for their productivity, their ability to withstand mechanical picking and cross-country shipping, and their tolerance of pesticides. With less biodiversity the chances of catastrophic crop failures increase.

Two of the better known benefits of heirloom seed include adaptability and flavor. Some varieties of heirloom tomato have been known to adapt to a specific location within as little as 2 to 3 growing seasons, showing better vigor, better production, better flavor and increased disease resistance. This is a result of saving the seed and replanting it year to year.

The definition and use of the word heirloom to describe plants is fiercely debated.

My idea of what an heirloom seed is: it has never been cross pollinated, it has never been hybrid and it has never been genetically modified. If there is a crop of Heirloom plants in one field and plants of another variety in an adjacent field and they cross pollinate the resulting plant is something other than heirloom.

Most heirlooms have been saved and selected because they have the best flavor and production in home and small market gardens. We get the benefit of this long development cycle, as only the best producing, most flavorful, most memorable and most dependable varieties have made the selection throughout the years. Delicate, weak or fickle varieties are no longer with us.

Open-pollinated is a term sometimes used interchangeably with heirloom. The terms actually have different meanings, as an open pollinated seed is simply a variety where the seed can be harvested from the plant, saved, replanted, and the same variety will re-grow year after year. All heirloom seeds are open pollinated; open pollinated seeds *may be* heirloom, as there are new open pollinated varieties being introduced that are obviously too recent to be considered heirlooms and sometimes are the result of cross pollination. A problem with the term "open-pollination" is that some of these crops have no seeds, and no pollination, open or otherwise is required to keep these varieties going. Potatoes, garlic, Jerusalem artichokes and certain others are propagated vegetatively. Calling such crops "open-pollinated" *feels* awkward, even if such cultivars first grew from seed.

Adapted by author from many sources beginning in 2001 before I knew I would be writing this book.

Hybrid Plants And Animals

A **hybrid** seed is produced by artificially cross pollinating two genetically different plants of the same species, such as two different tomatoes or two varieties of corn. The cross pollination is done by hand, and a seed that is saved will have a different genetic makeup than either parent. Hybrids are typically bred for commercial use and profit. The changes to the characteristic of the resulting plants are to increase yield, uniformity, more even ripening, improved color and disease resistance. Flavor has only recently begun to be addressed when selecting characteristics for new hybrids.

Hybrids originated in the 1920s and 1930s for small local commercial growers who shipped their produce less than 50 miles to market, and needed more consistent production for a steady supply of fresh produce to the markets. Hybrids of today are selected primarily for looks and being able to withstand shipping long distances. This has resulted in the iconic colorful yet flavorless supermarket tomato that looks and tastes the same year round and is less nutritious.

Hybrids are developed by mating two species, normally from within the same genus. The offspring display traits and characteristics of both parents.

As an example almost all apple trees are hybrids in an attempt to combine the best characteristics of two different apples.

Adapted by author from many sources beginning in 2001 before I knew I would be writing this book.

GMO Foods

What Are GMO Foods?

There is quite a bit of concern regarding GMO foods in our country. With 50 or so countries requiring labeling or restrictions on genetically modified foods, it is curious as to why we allow inadequate and misleading labeling? How come Russia, China, New Zealand, Taiwan, Chile, South Africa, Japan, Brazil, and many others, find these ingredients to be problematic, and possibly detrimental to public health?

Genetically Modified Organisms, or GMOs, are organisms that have had specific variables introduced into their DNA by mans manipulation. These variables are foreign to them. These variables may help reduce pests, or create frost-free varieties of certain vegetables. I question the consequences of tinkering with nature and introducing new manipulated GMO foods into our food supply.

There is evidence that instead of reducing pests the tinkering instead creates super pests.

There is already quite a bit of evidence piling up on the health effects of these unnatural "foods". Fertility issues are one of the problems associated with the consumption of GMOs, as well as cancer, diabetes, Alzheimer's, and even gluten-intolerance.

Adapted by author from <http://articles.mercola.com/sites/articles/archive/2011/10/06/dangerous-toxins-from-gmo-foods.aspx>

GMO Is No Longer Just For Foods (sometimes called GE)

Monsanto and Scotts have begun testing the first genetically engineered (GE) grass, intended for both consumer and commercial use.

Scotts Roundup-Ready Kentucky Bluegrass, genetically engineered to withstand massive amounts of Monsanto's Roundup herbicide, is unregulated, will **not** be labeled "GMO" (genetically modified organisms), and because of the ease with which grass spreads, could in short order contaminate lawns, parks, golf courses and pastures everywhere.

Because Roundup will kill everything except the grass engineered to stand up to it, lawns all over the country will be green, lush—and toxic.

And you wo**n't** know it.

"As these seeds spread and more and more grass takes up that genetic trait, we'll find organic farmers who want to grass feed their beef, ca**n't** do it because their grass is genetically modified, which is prohibited in organic standards," said Bill Duesing of the Northeast Organic Farming Association, in an article in *CT News Junkie*. "GMOs are pollution with a life of its own."

In July 2011, Scotts Company and Monsanto convinced the U.S. Department of Agriculture (USDA) to give the companies a free pass to market Roundup-Ready Kentucky Bluegrass. No testing required.

How did they circumvent the system? GE crops are regulated by the USDA under rules pertaining to plant pests. These rules were created in the 1950s to give the USDA some muscle to constrain the introduction of organisms that would inflict harm to plants. Because genetically modified crops use DNA material derived from natural plant pathogens, they technically qualify as "plant pests."

Scotts got around this level of restriction because they avoided using plant pests in the development of the Kentucky Bluegrass. Instead, the glyphosate-resistant gene originated from other plants that were **not** considered pathogens. Furthermore, the gene was fired in with a gene gun, instead of being carried by a plant pest bacterium. By avoiding the use of plant pests in the engineering process, Scotts has also avoided that regulation trigger.

The second mechanism the USDA could have used to regulate GMO grass is the noxious weed provision under the Plant Protection Act of 2000. It's well known that bluegrass spreads easily, because its light pollen can be carried for miles on the wind. Inevitably, genetically modified bluegrass will transfer its genes to established conventional bluegrass.

That's one reason Scotts Roundup-Ready grass is so dangerous—it threatens to contaminate every lawn, park, roadside and field in sight, including the pastures used by organic farmers to graze their cattle. This puts organic farmers at risk of losing their certification and it puts the animals at risk of eating GMO grass. Research shows that GMO grain has a devastating impact on the health of animals raised for slaughter. Will GMO grass also be hazardous to animal health, including cattle raised for meat—and people's prized horses?

Beyond its ability to spread quickly, beyond its potential impact on organic farmers, even more troubling is the fact that once Scotts Roundup Ready grass hits the market, it will lead to a dramatic increase in the use of Roundup. Roundup is already the most widely used, and potentially the most harmful, herbicide in the world.

And much of that Roundup will be lurking in places where kids play.

Glyphosate, the active ingredient in Roundup herbicide has recently been described by researchers as, "the most biologically disruptive chemical in our environment." It's been linked to a litany of health disorders and diseases including Parkinson's, cancer and autism.

Studies have revealed a connection between the use of glyphosate and birth defects in frog and chicken embryos. A more recent study shows that the toxic herbicide was found in the breast milk of American women.

This month (May 2014), employees of Scotts begin testing the new product at their homes. Scotts' CEO told shareholders his goal is to have the GMO ready for commercial applications in 2015, and on the consumer market in 2016.

Scotts, which is Monsanto's exclusive agent for the marketing and distribution of consumer Roundup, has much to gain by releasing its frankengrass into the marketplace. According to *The Columbus Dispatch*, CEO Hagedorn in January told shareholders the market opportunity for Roundup-Ready Bluegrass is substantial. "If you look at the grass-seed category, it's probably significantly north of $500 million and probably less than $1 billion."

The company is determined to protect its projected revenue. When Connecticut came close to passing a statewide ban on GMO grass, Hagedorn reportedly sent a letter to Gov. Dannel Malloy (D-CT) stating that any renewed effort to ban or place a moratorium on the new seed could result in Hagedorn questioning "whether continuing to invest in Connecticut is in the best long-term interests of my company and its stockholders."

Monsanto and Scotts are both members of the **Grocery Manufacturers Association**, which has spent millions to defeat GMO labeling laws and bans, and plans to sue Vermont to overturn its recently passed law requiring mandatory labeling of foods containing GMOs. The Organic Consumers Association has called for a boycott of all products marketed by members of the Grocery Manufacturers Association.

We also urge consumers everywhere to contact Hagedorn and other executives at Scotts to inform them that they will boycott all Scotts products unless the company drops plans to market its Roundup-Ready Kentucky Bluegrass.

By Charlotte Warren: a communications consultant to the Organic Consumers Association.

and Ronnie Cummins: the national director for the Organic Consumers Association.

Adapted by author from <http://gmofreeplanet.com/uncategorized/gmo-grass-coming-lawn-near> May 22, 2014

Bt-Toxin produced in GM corn and cotton plants

There's already plenty of evidence that the Bt-toxin produced in GM corn and cotton plants is toxic to humans and mammals *and* triggers immune system responses. The fact that it flows through our blood supply and that it passes through the placenta into fetuses, may help explain the rise in many disorders in the US since Bt crop varieties were first introduced in 1996.

In government sponsored research in Italy, mice fed Monsanto's Bt corn showed a wide range of immune responses. Their elevated IgE and IgG antibodies, for example, are typically associated with allergies and infections. The mice had an increase in cytokines, which are associated with "allergic and inflammatory responses." The specific cytokines (interleukins) that were elevated are also higher in humans who suffer from a wide range of disorders, from arthritis and inflammatory bowel disease, to MS and cancer (see chart).

Elevated interleukins	Associations
IL-6	Rheumatoid arthritis, inflammatory bowel disease, osteoporosis, multiple sclerosis, various types of cancer (multiple myeloma and prostate cancer)
IL-13	Allergy, allergic rhinitis, ALS (Lou Gehrig's disease)
MIP-1b	Autoimmune disease and colitis
IL-12p70	Inflammatory bowel disease, multiple sclerosis

The young mice in the study also had elevated T cells (gamma delta), which are increased in people with asthma, and in children with food allergies, juvenile arthritis and connective tissue diseases. The Bt corn that was fed to these mice, MON 810, produced the same Bt-toxin that was found in the blood of women and fetuses.

When rats were fed another of Monsanto's Bt corn varieties called MON 863, their immune systems were also activated, showing higher numbers of basophils, lymphocytes, and white blood cells. These can indicate possible allergies, infections, toxins, and various disease states including cancer. There were also signs of toxicity in the liver and kidneys.

Bt-Toxin Is Dangerous

Farmers have used Bt-toxin from soil bacteria as a natural pesticide for years. **But** they *spray* it on plants, where it washes off and biodegrades in sunlight. The GM version is built-in; every plant cell has its own spray bottle. The toxin stays in the GMO food no matter how much it rains or how well you wash it off. The Bt-toxin is consumed with the food. Furthermore, the plant-produced version of the poison in GMO crops is thousands of times more concentrated than the spray, is designed to be even more toxic and has properties of known allergens. It actually *fails* the World Health Organization's allergen screening tests.

When *natural* Bt-toxin was fed to mice, they had tissue damage, immune responses as powerful as cholera toxin and even started reacting to other foods that were formerly harmless. Farm workers exposed to Bt also showed immune responses. The EPA's own expert Scientific Advisory Panel said that these mouse and farm worker studies "suggest that Bt proteins could act as antigenic and allergenic sources. **But** the EPA ignored the warnings. They also overlooked studies showing that about 500 people in Washington state and Vancouver showed allergic and flu-like symptoms when they were exposed to the spray when it was used to kill gypsy moths.

Glyphosate Toxicity—Another Hidden Danger Of GE Foods

There's also another potent toxin associated with genetically engineered foods that is unrelated to the Bt toxin or the genetic alteration itself, and that is glyphosate - the active ingredient in Monsanto's broad-spectrum herbicide, which is used on both GE crops and many conventional crops as well. The contamination appears to be greater in GE crops however, especially in so-called Roundup Ready crops. These are genetically altered to withstand otherwise lethal doses of the herbicide, and it's important to realize that the glyphosate *permeates the entire plant*. It is impossible to wash off

In June, groundbreaking research was published detailing a newfound mechanism of harm for Roundup. The finding suggests that glyphosate may actually be *the most important factor* in the development of a wide variety of chronic diseases, specifically because your gut bacteria are a key component of glyphosate's mechanism of harm.

Monsanto has steadfastly claimed that Roundup is harmless to animals and humans because the mechanism of action it uses (which allows it to kill weeds), called the shikimate pathway, is absent in all animals. What they fail to mention is that the shikimate pathway IS present in bacteria, and that's the key to understanding how it causes such widespread systemic harm in both humans and animals. The bacteria in your body outnumber your cells by 10 to 1. For every cell in your body, you have 10 microbes of various kinds, and all of them have the shikimate pathway, so they will *all* respond to the presence of glyphosate!

Glyphosate causes extreme disruption of the microbe's function and lifecycle. What's worse, glyphosate *preferentially* affects *beneficial* bacteria, allowing pathogens to overgrow and take over. At that point, your body also has to contend with the toxins produced by the pathogens. Once the chronic inflammation sets in, you're well on your way toward chronic and potentially debilitating disease.

Roundup is actually patented as a biocide. It's an antibiotic; it kills bacteria. It kills the beneficial bacteria that provide the nutrients to the soil. It also kills the beneficial bacteria in your gut... It kills the Bifidus. It kills the Lactobacillus. When you kill the beneficial gut bacteria, it affects your immune system and digestive tract. It keeps alive the E.coli, salmonella, botulism and other agents of disease.

This remarkable finding was immediately followed by tests showing that people in 18 countries across Europe have glyphosate in their bodies, while yet another study revealed that the chemical has estrogenic properties and drives breast cancer proliferation in the parts-per-*trillion* range. This finding might help explain why rats fed Monsanto's maize (corn) developed massive breast tumors in the first-ever lifetime feeding study published.

Other recently published studies demonstrate glyphosate's toxicity to cell lines, aquatic life, food animals and humans. In fact, research has shown that Roundup is toxic to human DNA even when diluted to concentrations 450-fold lower than used in agricultural applications. Liver, embryonic, and placental cell lines are adversely affected by glyphosate at doses as low as 1 ppm. GMO corn can contain as much as 13 ppm of glyphosate, and Americans eat an average of 193 lbs of GMO foods annually.

Avoid processed foods of all kinds, as they're virtually guaranteed to contain genetically engineered ingredients, and center your diet around whole, organic foods as toxic pesticides are prohibited in organic farming. Supporting GMO labeling is also important in order to be able to make informed shopping decisions.

Adapted by author from
<http://articles.mercola.com/sites/articles/archive/2011/10/06/dangerous-toxins-from-gmo-foods.aspx>

Personal Notes

Common GMO Foods

Also check labels for any ingredients using these as an ingredient.
Examples: 'Corn Syrup' is made from corn, 'Soy Protein' is made from soy.

Main GMO Foods	Comment
Apples	First GMO apple awaiting approval as of December 2013.It will retain its pretty color when sliced.
Canola (Rapeseed) Oil (80% GMO))	GMO FOOD - Canola is genetically modified rapeseed (used to make mustard gas), designed to be resistant to Monsanto's Round Up herbicide. One possible effect of long-term use is the destruction of the protective coating surrounding nerves called the myelin sheath. This is like having raw, open wires in the body.
Corn (85% GMO)	GMO FOOD - Modified to create its own insecticide.
Cotton (88% GMO)	GMO FOOD - Modified to resist pesticides. It is considered food because its oil can be consumed
Dairy Products	GMO FOOD - Cows are injected with recombinant (genetically modified) bovine growth hormone (rBGH). Also fed GMO feeds.
Golden Rice	GMO FOOD -
Honey	Honey can be produced from GM crops. Some Canadian honey comes from bees collecting nectar from GM canola plants. This has shut down exports of Canadian honey to Europe.
Meat	Meat, dairy and farm raised fish products usually come from animals that have eaten GM feed
Papaya (50% GMO)	GMO FOOD - Modified to be resistant to the Papaya Ringspot Virus. More than 50% of the papaya crops in the US (including Hawaiian) are modified.
Peas	GMO FOOD - A gene from kidney beans was inserted into the peas creating a protein that functions as a pesticide.
Potatoes	GMO FOOD - Engineered with Bacillus thuringiensis
Rice	GMO FOOD - This staple food from South East Asia has now been genetically modified to contain a high amount of vitamin A.

Main GMO Foods	Comment
Farm Raised Fish	GMO FOOD - Some are GMO and some are fed GMO foods.
Soy (91% GMO)	GMO FOOD - Modified to resist herbicides. Soy products include soy flour, tofu, soy beverages, soybean oil and other products that include soy.
Sugar Beets (95% GMO)	GMO FOOD - Engineered to be resistant to certain pesticides and able to tolerate heavy pesticide crop spray.
Sugar Cane	GMO FOOD - Engineered to be resistant to certain pesticides and able to tolerate heavy pesticide crop spray.
Tomatoes (first GMO food)	GMO FOOD - Engineered to extend shelf life
Zucchini And Yellow Squash	GMO FOOD - Closely related, these two squash varieties are modified to resist viruses.
Aspartame	GMO FOOD - Aspartame is a toxic additive used in numerous food products, and should be avoided for numerous reasons, including the fact that it is created with genetically modified bacteria.
Tobacco	The company Vector has a GMO tobacco being sold under the brand of Quest® cigarettes in the U.S. It is engineered to produce low or no nicotine.
Vitamins	Vitamin C (ascorbic acid) is often made from corn, vitamin E is usually made from soy. Vitamins A, B2, B6, and B12 may be derived from GMOs. Vitamin D and vitamin K may have "carriers" derived from GM corn sources, such as starch, glucose, and maltodextrin. At least one Omega 3 and 6 supplement is made with GMO algae and GMO soil fungus.
Always check labels for these ingredients and avoid unless its organic: 1) Canola 2) anything with the word Corn 3) anything with the word Cottonseed 4) any Dairy product 5) Honey 6) any meat 7) Papaya 8) Peas 9) Patatoes 10) Rice 11) sugar 12) Zucchini 13) Yellow Squash 14) Vitamins	

The table above was created by the author from his own research.

GMO Companies

Companies That Use GMO Foods and Are Fighting Against The Labeling Initiatives

Companies Donating to Fight GMO Labeling in Washington State	Amount Donated	Comment
Abbott Nutrition	$127,459	
Basf Plant Science		Hide GMO and Contribute Hidden Money
Bayer Cropscience		Hide GMO and Contribute Hidden Money
Bimbo Bakeries Usa	$94,693	
Biotechnology Industry Org.		Biotech GMO Company that Contributed $
Bruce Foods Corp.	$3,006	
Bumble Bee Foods	$36,073	
Bunge North America	$94,993	
Bush Brothers & Co.	$16,233	
C. H. Guenther & Son, Inc.		Hide GMO and Contribute Hidden Money
Campbell Soup Co.	$265,140	
Cargill Inc.	$98,601	
Clement Pappas & Co. Inc	$21,043	
Clorox Company	$12,024	
Coca-Cola	$1,047,332	
Conagra Foods	$285,281	
Council For Biotechnology Information		Biotech GMO Company that Contributed $
Dean Foods	$120,245	
Del Monte Foods	$86,576	
Dole Packaged Foods Company		Hide GMO and Contribute Hidden Money
Dow Agrosciences LLC		Biotech GMO Company that Contributed $
E.I. DuPont De Nemours & Co.		Biotech GMO Company that Contributed $
FirstVote Pac		Biotech GMO Company that Contributed $
Flowers Foods	$141,288	
Gatorade		Use hidden GMO foods in their products
General Mills	$598,819	
Godiva Chocolatier, Inc.		Hide GMO and Contribute Hidden Money
Grocery Manufacturers Association		Biotech GMO Assosiation that Contributed $
Hero North America		Hide GMO and Contribute Hidden Money
Hershey	$248,305	
Hillshire Brands	$97,398	
Companies Donating to Fight GMO Labeling in Washington State	Amount Donated	Comment

Hormel Foods	$52,908	
House-Autry Mills, Inc.		Hide GMO and Contribute Hidden Money
Inventure Foods, Inc.		Hide GMO and Contribute Hidden Money
J.M. Smucker Co	$241,091	
Kellogg	$221,852	
Knouse Foods Cooperative Inc.	$14,429	
Kraft		Hide GMO and Contribute Hidden Money
Labatt beer		Use hidden GMO foods in their products
Land O'lakes	$99,803	
Mars Food North America		Hide GMO and Contribute Hidden Money
Mccain Foods Usa, Inc.		Hide GMO and Contribute Hidden Money
Mccormick & Co	$102,208	
Miss Vickie's		Use hidden GMO foods in their products
Mondelez Global	$144,895	
Moody Dunbar	$1,804	
Morton Salt		Hide GMO and Contribute Hidden Money
Nestle USA	$1,052,743	
Ocean Spray, Cranberries, Inc.	$55,313	
Oregonians For Food And Shelter		Biotech GMO Company that Contributed $
Pepsico (PEPSICO, INC.)	$1,620,899	
Pinnacle Foods Group	$120,846	Hide GMO and Contribute Hidden Money
President's Choice		Use hidden GMO foods in their products
Quaker Oats		Use hidden GMO foods in their products
Ragu		Use hidden GMO foods in their products
Rich Products Corp	$24,049	Biotech GMO Company that Contributed $
Sara Lee Corporation		Hide GMO and Contribute Hidden Money
Shearer's Foods, Inc.	$25,251	
Solae, LLC		Hide GMO and Contribute Hidden Money
Sunny Delight Beverages Co.	$21,043	
Syngenta Corporation		Biotech GMO Company that Contributed $
Welch Foods	$28,859	
Wm. Wrigley Jr. Company		Hide GMO and Contribute Hidden Money

The table above was created by the author from his own research.

Genetically Modified Soil Fungus and Algae
In Organic Foods And Baby Formula

The following information on GMO soil fungus and algae used as a food supplement is Adapted by author from Dr. Mercola's information rich website: <mercola.com>

By Dr. Mercola

Last December (2011), the U.S. National Organic Standards Board, an expert panel that advises the USDA Secretary on organic matters, narrowly approved Martek Biosciences Corporation's petition to allow the use of their genetically modified soil fungus and algae as nutritional supplements in organic food.

The product is an omega-3/omega-6 oil (DHA/ARA) synthesized from fermented algae and soil fungus.

The oil is extracted from this biomass using hexane, a neurotoxic byproduct of gasoline refinement that is specifically banned in organics.

The Cornucopia Institute investigated Martek's patent and safety filings at the FDA, and discovered that the product also contains synthetic chemicals, stabilizers, carriers, and some of the ingredients are also genetically modified.

(As it turns out, some of Martek's products were developed by Monsanto before Martek bought the technical rights.)

Martek's formulated oils are added to "organic" milk, infant formula, and a number of different foods. After a formal legal complaint, the USDA announced in 2010 that it had "inappropriately" allowed Martek oils to be included in organic foods.

But enforcement of their removal was delayed for 18 months in an apparent effort to permit corporate lobbyists to petition for review and legal inclusion in organic food. According to the Conucopia Institute:

"Although Martek told the board that they would discontinue the use of the controversial neurotoxic solvent n-hexane for DHA/ARA processing, they withheld what other synthetic solvents would be substituted. Federal organic standards prohibit the use of all synthetic/petrochemical solvents."

How Did Unapproved Ingredients Make it into Baby Food?

It is distressing to see that chemical additives have skirted USDA approval and made their way into infant formulas – some of which even bear the USDA Organic Seal! This confirms that even organic certification leaves room for interpretation, and you, the consumer, will need to stay on your toes.

Martek's DHA and ARA products are synthetic attempts at omega-3 fats that have been in the U.S. marketplace since 2002, and in organic products since 2006. They are chemically extracted from certain types of algae and fungi that have never before been part of the human diet, and have never been approved by the USDA. Yet they have made their way into your baby's bottle.

In fact, it is unlikely that the production process of these agents has been examined at all – and for good reason. The Cornucopia Institute has uncovered an entire list of questions regarding the source, processing, and other ingredients used in the manufacturing of Martek's DHA and ARA, any one of which could result in a ban from their use in certified organic products.

GMOs, Lies, and Petrochemicals

For starters, Martek's synthetic oils are extracted using a toxic petrochemical solvent called hexane – a process that's just about as NON-organic as you can get. Hexane extraction is widely used in the production of oils, such as fatty acids and vegetable oils, **but** is banned in organic produce because it's a non-organic material.

So what's their loophole?

Martek Biosciences was able to dodge the ban on hexane-extraction by claiming the USDA considers omega-3 and omega-6 fats to be "necessary vitamins and minerals," instead of "agricultural ingredients." Therefore, they argue, the ban against hexane extraction is invalid. The USDA helped them out by classifying those oils as "necessary vitamins and minerals," which are exempt from the hexane ban. **But** hexane-extraction is just the tip of the iceberg. Other questionable manufacturing practices and misleading statements by Martek include:

> Undisclosed synthetic ingredients, prohibited for use in organics (including the sugar alcohol mannitol, modified starch, glucose syrup solids, and "other" undisclosed ingredients)

> Microencapsulation of the powder and nanotechnology, which are prohibited under organic laws

> Use of volatile synthetic solvents, besides hexane (such as isopropyl alcohol)

> Recombinant DNA techniques and other forms of genetic modification of organisms; mutagenesis; use of GMO corn as a fermentation medium

> Heavily processed ingredients that are far from "natural"

Your Body Knows These "Nutrients" Are Fake

Although DHA and ARA from real foods are indeed important nutrients, the synthetic versions are far from being the same. They are foreign to your body, and to your infant's body, which is why many babies are having terrible adverse reactions. Naturally derived omega-3 fats have important benefits to your baby's eyes and brain. Martek has manipulated this fact into a clever marketing ploy that convinces mothers that this artificial concoction is as good for their babies as breast milk.

There is no scientific evidence to substantiate Martek's health claims. Martek claims that their formula is "proven in independent clinical studies to enhance mental development." According to the Cornucopia Institute, this claim is based on one single study involving just 19 infants. Martek neglects to mention the numerous other clinical studies that fail to show any advantage in brain development.

The Perfect Formula For Diarrhea, Vomiting And Gastrointestinal Pain

The Cornucopia Institute has compiled a summary of hundreds of adverse reports submitted to the FDA about possible intolerance to DHA/ARA-supplemented infant formula. Of those reports, 98 are said to be "confidently linked" to intolerance to the DHA/ARA oils. Many hundreds more are highly suspect. The reported gastrointestinal symptoms include:

Severe gas

Diarrhea and vomiting

Gastric reflux

Constipation and bowel obstruction

Agitation, fussiness, crying, and severe distress

The adverse reaction reports filed with the FDA represent only the tip of the iceberg, as most parents are unaware that Martek's additives may be the cause of their infants' problems. Some parents and their babies have endured these symptoms for weeks or months before identifying the cause, believing it was simply colic or unexplained fussiness.

A few companies have made a conscious decision to leave Martek's additives out of their baby food products, in order to protect the organic integrity of their foods. Cornucopia has published a list of "USDA Organic" products containing Martek's additives. Shockingly, ALL organic infant formulas with the exception of ONE (Baby's Only Organic) contain Martek's DHA! Some baby foods also contain it, so it's a good idea to get in the habit of reading ALL of your labels.

Adapted by author from <http://articles.mercola.com/sites/articles/archive/2012/04/01/gmo-infant-formula.aspx>

Livestock And Animal Feed Additives

I have removed Dr. Mercola's footnotes from this section. Please go to the original articles listed in the references to access his sources.

By Dr. Mercola

Meat—and beef in particular—is a mainstay of the traditional American dinner. Unfortunately, the vast majority of it is filled with harmful additives of one form or another, and is raised in such a way that it contributes to the *degeneration* of health...

This is no minor concern, as most of the animals are also fed genetically engineered feed that is loaded with the potent herbicide glyphosate that winds up in your body.

I am so convinced of the cumulative harms of consuming meat from animals raised in confined animal feeding operations (CAFO's) that the ONLY type of meat I recommend eating (and the only meat I will eat myself) is organically-raised, grass-fed or pastured meats and animal byproducts.

This applies to <u>all types of meat: beef, pork and poultry, including turkey</u>.

(Glenn's comment: This also applies to farm raised fish).

In a recent article published by the Cornucopia Institute, investigative health reporter Martha Rosenberg discusses the questionable yet widespread use of Ractopamine in American animal farming.

Ractopamine

According to Rosenberg, the controversial drug is used in as many as 80 percent of all American pig and cattle operations. It's also used in turkey farming.

FDA Sued for Withholding Records Pertaining to Ractopamine Safety

Ractopamine is a beta agonist drug that increases protein synthesis, thereby making the animal more muscular. This reduces the fat content of the meat and increases the profit per animal. The drug, which is also used in asthma medication, was initially recruited for use in livestock when researchers discovered that it made mice more muscular.

Interestingly enough, stubborn weight gain is also common complaint among asthma patients using Advair (a beta-agonist drug)—so much so that the manufacturer has added weight gain to the post-marketing side effects. Other adverse reactions to beta-agonist drugs include increased heart rate, insomnia, headaches and tremors.

Beta-agonist drugs, as a class, have been used in US cattle production since 2003. The drug is administered in the days leading up to slaughter, and as much as 20 percent of it can remain in the meat you buy.

This is disconcerting when you consider that the drug label warns: "**Not** for use in humans," and "individuals with cardiovascular disease should exercise special caution to avoid exposure."

While other drugs require a clearance period of around two weeks to help ensure the compounds are flushed from the meat prior to slaughter (and therefore reduce residues leftover for human consumption), there is no clearance period for ractopamine.

In an effort to get this dangerous additive out of American meat products, the Center for Food Safety (CFS) and Animal Legal Defense Fund (ALDF) recently sued the US Food and Drug Administration (FDA) for withholding records pertaining to ractopamine's safety. As reported by Rosenberg:

> "According to the lawsuit, in response to the groups' requests for information "documenting, analyzing, or otherwise discussing the physiological, psychological, and/or behavioral effects" of ractopamine, the FDA has only produced 464 pages out of 100,000 pages that exist.

> Worse, all 464 pages have already been released as part of a reporter's FOIA...

> CFS and ALDF have spent over 18 months meeting with the FDA and seeking information about the effects of ractopamine on "target animal or human liver form and function, kidney form and function, thyroid form and function" as well as urethral and prostate effects and "tumor development." The lawsuit says the CFS has "exhausted administrative remedies" and that the FDA has "unlawfully withheld" the materials."

Why Is Ractopamine Banned In 160 Countries?

Ractopamine is banned from food production in at least 160 countries around the world, including countries across Europe, Russia, mainland China and Republic of China (Taiwan), due to its suspected health effects. Since 1998, more than 1,700 people have reportedly been "poisoned" from eating pigs fed the drug. If imported meat is found to contain traces of the drug, it is turned away, while fines and imprisonment result for its use in banned countries.

While Americans are largely unaware that the drug is even used, many other nations seem to be far better informed. Fear that the ractopamine ban might be lifted brought thousands of demonstrators onto the streets in Taiwan last year, demanding that the ban remain in place.

In February of this year, Russia issued a ban on US meat imports, warning it would remain in place until the US agrees to certify that the meat is ractopamine-free. As reported by Pravda, Russia is the fourth largest importer of US meats, purchasing about $500 million-worth of beef and pork annually. At present, in the US there is no testing for the presence of this drug in meats sold, even though animal research has linked ractopamine to:

1. Reductions in reproductive function
2. Birth defects (Canadian researchers found that, in rats, the drug produced a variety of birth defects, including cleft palate, protruding tongue, short limbs, missing or fused digits, open eyelids, jaw abnormalities, limb abnormalities, and enlarged heart)
3. Increase of mastitis (an infection of the breast tissue) in dairy herds
4. Increased disability and death

In both pigs and cattle, FDA reports link the drug to: excessive hunger, anorexia, bloat, respiratory and hoof problems, lameness, stiffness, stress and aggression, and—again—death. In fact, of all reported side effects, death topped the list as the most reported problem associated with ractopamine...

Ractopamine is also known to affect the human cardiovascular system, and is thought to be responsible for hyperactivity. It may also cause chromosomal abnormalities and behavioral changes. According to the Russian news source Pravda, the drug may cause food poisoning, and Center for Food Safety (CFS) states, "that data from the European Food Safety Authority indicates that ractopamine causes elevated heart rates and heart-pounding sensations in humans."

Two cousin drugs of ractopamine, clenbuterol and zilpaterol, cause such adrenalin effects in humans they are banned by the Olympics.

Roesenberg writes. "Cyclist Alberto Contador failed a Tour de France anti-doping test in 2010 for levels of clenbuterol which he said he got from eating meat. Clenbuterol has been banned or restricted in meat after human toxicities. "The use of highly active beta-agonists as growth promoters is inappropriate because of the potential hazard for human and animal health," wrote the journal Talanta. *"*

Zilmax - An Even More Dangerous Beta Agonist Drug Used In Livestock?

Zilmax (Zilpaterol) is another beta-agonist drug used in cattle to increase weight by as much as 30 pounds of lean meat per cow. The drug recently got a slew of bad press when, in the beginning of August, Tyson Foods Inc declared it would no longer buy Zilmax-fed cattle for slaughter, due to concerns over behavioral problems in some of the cattle. Zilmax is already banned for use in horses due to severe side effects, including muscle tremors and rapid heart rates that can last as long as two weeks after stopping the drug. It is logical to imagine similar problems might occur in cattle. Zilmax is actually about 125 times more potent than ractopamine, and according to a 2008 veterinary report, this may be why side effects were overlooked in connection with ractopamine studies.

Merck, the manufacturer of Zilmax, has no plans on discontinuing the product however. After responding to Tyson's decision by stating it would halt US and Canadian sales of Zilmax pending research and review, the company recently told Reuters that it is in fact pushing to bring the drug back to market, both in the US and Canada. The company says it stands behind the safety of the drug and is working on developing a quality control program to "ensure its proper use."

The problem though is that even with proper use you're likely to end up with drug-laced meat. According to Randox Food Diagnostics, which has created tests for Zilmax residue in beef, use of beta-agonists prior to slaughter is of particular concern "as this poses a risk to the consumer and may result in consumer toxicity." (Remember, Zilmax is about 125 times more potent than ractopamine, making this drug an even greater concern in the large scope of things.) Research findings to this effect include:

> A 2003 study in Analytica Chimica Acta: Residue behavior of Zilmax in urine, plasma, muscle, liver, kidney and retina of cattle and pig was assessed. Two heifers and 16 pigs were treated with Zilmax and slaughtered after withdrawal times varying from 1 to 10 days. The drug was detectable at each point of time examined in all matrices except plasma after a withdrawal period of 10 days. It's worth noting that in the US, the recommended market window is three to 10 days after discontinuing Zilmax

> A 2006 study on residues of Zilmax in sheep found detectable levels in liver and muscle tissues up to nine days after discontinuation of the drug

Do Beta-Agonists In Meat Pose Human Health Hazards?

According to an article published in the Journal of Animal Science in 1998, there's data on "human intoxication following consumption of liver or meat from cattle treated with beta-agonists." The authors write:

"The use of highly active beta-agonists as growth promoters is inappropriate because of the potential hazard for human and animal health, as was recently concluded at the scientific Conference on Growth Promotion in Meat Production (Nov. 1995, Brussels)."

Before it was approved for use in American livestock, scientists worried that *illegal* use of beta agonists could result in increased cardiovascular risk for consumers. Today we eat *legally* treated meat, since these drugs are approved and widely used. Should we be concerned about cardiovascular health risks from non-organic meat products? I *feel* it is imperative.

Glyphosate Contamination - Another Hidden Hazard In CAFO Meats

The true toxicity of glyphosate—the active ingredient in Monsanto's broad-spectrum herbicide Roundup—is becoming devastatingly clear, and it has far-reaching ramifications for the entire food system. Research published last year showed that Roundup is toxic to human DNA even when diluted to concentrations 450-fold lower than used in agricultural applications, and *e*thoxylated adjuvants in glyphosate-based herbicides have been found to be "active principles of human cell toxicity." Cell damage and even cell death can occur at the residual levels found on Roundup-treated food crops, and the chemical has also been found to have estrogenic effects.

The reason I bring this up here is because factory farmed animals are fed a diet primarily made up of grains like corn and soy—and those grains are likely to be contaminated with glyphosate. Once an animal has been raised on glyphosate-contaminated feed, its meat is bound to be of inferior quality. More so than any other contamination hazard, I believe glyphosate-contamination may be one of the most pressing concerns when it comes to eating CAFO meats and animal byproducts. Besides the potential for bioaccumulation of glyphosate, the chemical has a distinct adverse effect on the animal's gut bacteria, and hence its overall health.

Monsanto has steadfastly claimed that Roundup is harmless to animals and humans because the mechanism of action it uses (which allows it to kill weeds), called the shikimate pathway, is absent in all animals. However, the shikimate pathway IS present in bacteria, and that's the key to understanding how it causes such widespread systemic harm in both animals and humans.

Groundbreaking research published this past June suggests glyphosate may actually be *the most important factor* in the development of a wide variety of chronic diseases, specifically because your gut bacteria are a key component of glyphosate's mechanism of harm. The same applies to animals that eat feed contaminated with this agricultural chemical. If the animal is chronically ill, how beneficial can you expect its meat to be for your own health?

How To Protect Yourself And Your Family From Potentially Harmful Foods

If you live in the US, it's important to realize that antibiotics, pesticides, genetically engineered ingredients, herbicides like glyphosate, hormones, and countless other drugs—such as beta agonists discussed above—are allowed in your food. Most people make the mistake of thinking that "beef is beef," or that one slab of pork is no different from another, being unaware of the vast differences between factory farmed, so-called CAFO, meats, and meats from organically-raised pastured animals.

While pastured, grass-fed meats and animal products are typically nutritionally superior, it's perhaps what these meats are free of that can have the greatest impact on your health and your family's health—especially your children, since we're then talking about the cumulative effect over a lifetime, including the developmental stages.

Growth-promoting drugs, hormones, antibiotics and feed with genetically engineered ingredients are prohibited for use in organically-raised animals. The feed prohibited includes GMO corn and soy and feed that has been treated with any pesticide. In short, organic foods are FAR "cleaner" in terms of additives and contaminations, and that applies across the board, from fruits and vegetables to animal products.

It all boils down to this: if you want to optimize your health, you must return to the basics of healthy food choices. If you want to avoid these questionable drugs and other potentially harmful ingredients permitted in the US food supply, then ditching processed foods is your best option. Put your focus on WHOLE organic foods -- foods that are unprocessed or altered from their original state -- food that has been grown or raised as nature intended, without the use of chemical additives, drugs, hormones, pesticides and fertilizers. This is the answer to a vast majority of our current health crises.

It is an easier task than it may seem to find a local farmer that can supply your family with healthy, humanely raised animal products and produce. At *LocalHarvest.org*, for instance, you can enter your zip code and find farmers' markets, family farms, and other sources of sustainably grown food in your area, all with the click of a button. Once you make the switch from supermarket to local farmer or your own garden, the choice will seem natural, and you can have peace of mind that the food you're feeding your family is as safe as possible.

Adapted by author from <http://articles.mercola.com/sites/articles/archive/2013/12/24/ractopamine-beta-agonist-drug.aspx> and from <http://articles.mercola.com/sites/articles/archive/2012/06/05/artificial-growth-hormones-affects-food.aspx>

rBGH Hormones

The following information on rBGH Hormones is adapted by author from Dr. Mercola's information rich website: <mercola.com>

By Dr. Mercola

Five years ago Robyn O'Brien was an average American mom; busy with four kids, living on a limited budget, and totally uninterested in hearing anyone lecture her about what to feed her kids. Then one day, after being served a typical breakfast consisting of Eggo waffles, blue-colored yoghurt and scrambled eggs, her youngest child suddenly had an acute allergic reaction. That very day, Robyn threw herself into researching food allergies, and virtually overnight, Robyn became a real-food activist.

She quickly learned that the foods sold in our grocery stores are often unsafe. On the contrary, many, and maybe most of them, now contain "foreign" ingredients that have never been tested for safety and are anything **but** natural. This includes the 'natural' ingredients.

That something has gone awry is obvious when you take a look at the statistics. Between 1997 and 2002 the number of peanut allergies doubled, and the number of hospitalizations related to allergic reactions to food increased by a whopping 265 percent. One out of 17 children now has some form of food allergy. And allergy rates have been rising.

When you consider that a food allergic reaction occurs when your body reacts to a food protein as *a foreign invader* (just like a virus or bacteria) which triggers an inflammatory response, the obvious question then becomes:

Is There Something New And "Foreign" In Our Food Today?

Absolutely!

Processed foods in general can contribute to allergies for a number of different reasons. Most processed foods contain a variety of food colorings, flavors, preservatives, and other additives can have a major impact. **But** there's another, even more insidious hazard lurking in American food stores...

In the mid-1990's, new food proteins were engineered and introduced into our food supply, yet many people are still, to this day, clueless about this. As O'Brien states, it was clearly done to maximize profitability for the food industry, yet NO human trials were ever conducted to see if these genetically engineered proteins were actually safe for animal - and human - consumption.

One of the first foods to undergo this change was milk, which incidentally is also the number one food allergen in the US.

In 1994, the dairy industry started using a genetically engineered growth hormone, rBGH (recombinant bovine growth hormone) on cows in order to increase milk production. However, it resulted in higher rates of disease in the treated livestock. To counteract the ill effects, dairies also had to start using more antibiotics, which we now know is one of the driving factors behind the rise in antibiotic-resistant superbugs in humans.

While Canada, the UK, Australia, New Zealand and 27 countries in Europe refused to use rBGH due to the fact that it's safety is unproven, the United States took the opposite stance, and basically decided that until it had been proven dangerous, it would be allowed...

As inconceivable as it may seem, prior to rBGH being introduced into the milk - and every other conceivable dairy product - that millions of Americans consume every day, it had only been tested on 30 rats for 90 days!

Why You Should Be Concerned About rBGH In Your Milk

Samuel Epstein, MD, a scientist at the University of Illinois School of Public Health, is one of the top experts on cancer prevention. He is frequently called upon to advise Congress about things in our environment that may cause cancer, and he has written eight books, including two books on this particular topic *What's in Your Milk?*, and *Got (Genetically Engineered) Milk?*

In his books, Dr. Epstein explains that rBGH milk is "qualitatively and quantitatively different from natural milk," and is "supercharged with high levels of a natural growth factor (IGF-1), excess levels of which have been incriminated as major causes of breast, colon, and prostate cancers."

In addition to increased IGF-1 levels, other differences between rBGH milk and natural milk include:

Contamination of milk by the genetically modified hormone rBGH	Contamination by pus and antibiotics resulting from the high incidence of mastitis in rBGH-injected cows
Contamination with illegal antibiotics and drugs used to treat mastitis and other rBGH-induced disease	Increased concentration of the thyroid hormone enzyme thyroxin-5'-monodeiodinase
Increased concentration of long-chain and decreased concentration of short-chain fatty acids	A reduction in levels of the milk protein casein

Armed with these facts, O'Brien began researching cancer rates, and lo and behold, the United States has the highest rates of cancer of any country on the planet. According to the statistics she compiled, one in two men, and one in three women are expected to get cancer in their lifetime.

One in eight American women has breast cancer, and only one out of every 10 breast cancer cases is attributed to genetics.

Ninety percent are triggered by environmental factors.

Finding Food Grown The Way Nature Intended

If you want to optimize your health, it is vital for you and your family to return to the basics of healthy food choices and typically this includes buying your food from responsible, high-quality, sustainable sources. This will help you avoid virtually all of the problems previously discussed in this article.

This is why I encourage you to support the small family farms in your area, particularly *organic* farms that respect the laws of nature and use the relationships between animals, plants, insects, soil, water and habitat to create synergistic, self-supporting, non-polluting, GMO-free ecosystems.

You can do this by visiting the farm directly, if you have one nearby, or by taking part in farmer's markets and community-supported agriculture programs and food coops.

During summer in the United States, fresh produce and other wonderful whole foods grown with the laws of nature in mind are available in abundance. Here are some great resources to obtain wholesome food that supports you, animal welfare and the environment:

> **Alternative Farming Systems Information Center**, Community Supported Agriculture (CSA) <http://www.nal.usda.gov/afsic/pubs/csa/csa.shtml>
> **Farmers' Markets** -- A national listing of farmers' markets. <http://www.ams.usda.gov/AMSv1.0/farmersmarkets>
> **Local Harvest** -- This Web site will help you find farmers' markets, family farms, and other sources of sustainably grown food in your area where you can buy produce, grass-fed meats, and many other goodies. <http://www.localharvest.org/>
> **Eat Well Guide: Wholesome Food from Healthy Animals** -- The Eat Well Guide is a free online directory of sustainably raised meat, poultry, dairy, and eggs from farms, stores, restaurants, inns, and hotels, and online outlets in the United States and Canada. <http://www.eatwellguide.org/i.php?pd=Home>
> **Community Involved in Sustaining Agriculture** (CISA) -- CISA is dedicated to sustaining agriculture and promoting the products of small farms. <http://www.buylocalfood.org/>
> **FoodRoutes** -- The FoodRoutes "Find Good Food" map can help you connect with local farmers to find the freshest, tastiest food possible. On their interactive map, you can find a listing for local farmers, CSA's, and markets near you. <http://foodroutes.org/>

Adapted by author from <http://articles.mercola.com/sites/articles/archive/2013/12/24/ractopamine-beta-agonist-drug.aspx> and from <http://articles.mercola.com/sites/articles/archive/2012/06/05/artificial-growth-hormones-affects-food.aspx>

Mutagenesis

A form of genetically modifying plants that is unregulated and can be used in the production of "organic foods".

A method used in plant breeding whereby random mutations are induced in plant DNA using chemicals or ionising radiation. When a mutation is induced that is wanted (will increase profits) the 'food' is then marketed.

USDA Organic rules *do* allow mutagenesis in organic even though mutagenesis is a form of genetic modification.

Poisons And Toxins

A distinction between the two terms is debated, even among scientists. The closet consensus I could come up with follows.

Poison:

In the context of biology, poisons are substances that cause disturbances to organisms. The term poison is often used to describe any harmful substance, particularly corrosive substances, carcinogens, mutagens and harmful pollutants.

Toxin:

A substance that accumulates in the body and causes it harm. Toxins are poisons produced by some biological function in nature

To me whether something is called a poison or a toxin is unimportant. Does it harm the physical body or the environment?

Anything can be toxic in high enough doses and concentrations.

My question is it beneficial to plants, animals and the planet in appropriate quantities.

What is toxic to one species may be beneficial to another. Think of foods that are healthy and beneficial for some animals are deadly to others.

Food For Thought

Is Arsenic a poison/toxin?

Is 'Round Up' a poison/toxin?

Is bug spray to kill bugs a poison/toxin? Does it depend on the ingredients?

Is a bug repellent a poison/toxin? Does it depend on the ingredients?

Is vitamin D a poison/toxin? Does it depend on whether it is natural or synthetic?

Is a vitamin B shot a poison/toxin? Does it depend on whether it is natural or synthetic?

Is an injection of morphine a poison/toxin?

Is High Fructose Corn Syrup a poison/toxin?

Is water a poison/toxin?

Is GMO food a poison/toxin?

All substances can be toxic if too much is absorbed, breathed in, ingested or injected. Which of the above do you consider toxic or possibly toxic with no healthful benefits. Some seem clear and others take discernment and awareness of the ingredients.

Xenohormones And Estrogen Dominance

Xenohormones And Xenoestrogens

Xenohormones and Xenoestrogens affect Men, Women and Children. Xenohormones also spelled xeno-hormones and sometimes called xenoestrogens are a category of EDC's (Endocrine Disrupting Compounds) that are industrially made chemical compounds which disrupt communication within the bodies' endocrine/ hormone producing organs. These compounds have a negative estrogenic effect that differs chemically from naturally occurring hormones produced by living organisms.

Xenohormones are a group of manmade laboratory synthesized chemicals that are hormonally active agents that differ from phytoestrogens (estrogenic substances from plants), and can be divided into pharmacological estrogens and agents that have an unintended detrimental estrogenic effect.

"Estrogen like" substances from a variety of sources may have a cumulative effect upon living organisms. Xenohormones and xenoestrogens may be part of a larger picture of a process of estrogenisation of the environment we live in. The term estrogen dominance is used in some circles today which attribute these research findings to symptoms of estrogenisation displayed by women and men, child and adolescent.

Xenoestrogens and xenohormones have been introduced into the environment by industrial, agricultural and chemical companies in the last several decades. Their potential ecological and human health impact is under study and is of great concern to endocrinologists (specialist that study the hormone's and endocrine glands), environmentalist, scientists and doctors who see the hormone disruption caused by the confusion these chemicals cause when introduced into the biology of all living creatures.

A 2008 report demonstrates further evidence of wide-spread effects of feminizing chemicals on development in each class of vertebrate species as a worldwide phenomenon. Ninety-nine percent of over 100,000 recently introduced chemicals are poorly regulated and pose one of our civilizations greatest threats for survival.

Common Sources Of Xenohormones

Synthetic estrogens and progestins, as are found in oral contraceptives and conventional synthetic hormone replacement therapies.

All American-grown, non-organic livestock, which are fed estrogenic drugs to fatten them. Also, the grains they are fed are laden with chemical sprays that accumulate in animal tissue and promote hormone disruption in the person consuming them.

Petro chemically-derived pesticides, herbicides and fungicides. People use these in their gardens on their lawns and in the sprays they may use in their house or basement for pesky animals or mold growth.

The chemical Bisphenol A (also known as BPA), is used in plastic bottles, containers and almost all food-can liners. Very few states have restricted the use of this chemical and only when the community has banded together and petitioned the municipalities and local government has this been removed or restricted. The Food and Drug Administration will soon decide what it considers a safe level of exposure to Bisphenol A. Studies have already shown an increased incidence of breast and prostate cancers, diabetes and heart disease.

Solvents found in fingernail polish and polish remover, glue and cleaning supplies have been found to have the same cell proliferative properties and endocrine disruption.

Car exhaust is a real problem. If you live in a city or area where you are constantly exposed to this you should have a plan how to clear this from you system. Otherwise your doctor will be chasing symptoms with one diagnosis and drug to the next and next.

Emulsifiers found in soaps and cosmetics of the past and present are a real problem. Your skin being the largest organ is very capable of transferring chemicals through the membrane at a highly efficient rate, in most cases better than your gut. Find an organic source for this or one that you believe is the least harmful.

Almost all plastics, especially when plastics become hot or are heated. Studies have also shown that recycled plastics contain residues from their previous contents like dangerous herbicides, pesticides, poisons and chemical solvents. If you buy food that is stored or packaged in plastics, you are hoping that the plastic is harmless. Even in very small doses accumulated over time, these chemicals are harmful. A solution would be to transfer anything bought in plastic to something more stable, like a glass container.

Industrial wastes such as polychlorinated biphenyls (PCBs) and dioxins that may leak into the ground water and contaminate your drinking water. Have your tap water tested by a state agency to find out how many chemicals are found and what you can do to remove them.

Disorders and disease related to xenohormone exposure:

> Increase in reproductive-site cancers (breast, uterine, & ovarian)
> Decreased fertility in both male and females
> Estrogen dominance
> Increased incidence of prostate cancers
> Heart disease
> Diabetes type 2, adult onset
> Premature Ovarian Failure
> Uterine leiomyomas
> Prostate Cancer
> Obesity
> Thyroid Disruption
> Testicular Dysgensis Syndrome
> Endometriosis
> Uterine Fibroids

You can absorb xenohormones by ingestion, inhalation and direct skin contact. They exist in every aspect of your daily life; the coffee you drink from that Styrofoam cup, the fluorinated city water whether ingested or absorbed by your skin, the glue used in paper cups, the plastic alternative for your traveling mug and in the thermal paper used at nearly every store for your purchase receipt today. Xenohormones exist in the lining used on the inside of almost every can used for food found in your super market. To remove the sources of these endocrine disrupting agents you will have to search hard and remain diligent. Even your "safe" water supply contains chemicals meant to kill bacteria. These chemicals accumulate in our bodies and are now found in our ground water.

Our children also need to be protected from chlorinated pools, fluorinated drinking water, chlorinated tampons, shampoos, lipstick, hair spray, nail polish, perfumes and sodas in plastic containers. School foods that use government subsidized lunches from farms that use farming practices that produce unhealthy foods and are damaging to the environment have become the norm. These foods include meats laden with fattening chemical compounds found in all modern farming practices other than organic as well as GMO foods and foods designed to induce hunger and overeating.

What You Can Do To Minimize Xenohormone Exposure

Avoid all synthetic and horse hormones (oral contraceptives and conventional HRT).

Eat organic meat and dairy.

Avoid the fat of non-organic meat and dairy, including butter. This is where the greatest amount of unnatural hormones, pesticides, herbicides and other additives occurs and this is where xenohormones, xenoestrogens and endocrine disruptors will concentrate in non-organically raised livestock.

Decrease or stop all conventional pesticides, lawn and garden chemicals (use something natural instead). Avoid contracting with conventional lawn services that use these sprays (most do); they are extremely toxic and full of xenohormones and are endocrine disruptors.

Wear protective gloves and clothing when in contact with any glues, solvents or cleaning solutions that contain xenohormones.

Buy cosmetics without phthalates which are known xenohormones.

Avoid particle-board if you're remodeling or building a new house. Synthetic-fiber carpets and fake wood products are also loaded with known chemical disruptors.

Canned goods are almost always lined with Bisphenol A. Avoid as much as possible or transfer them to glass container or freeze them in the appropriate freezer bag.

Ventilate properly when in contact with any of these materials. Think ahead; for example, if you do install synthetic-fiber carpets, do so when the windows can be left open - it takes months to out-gas the chemical.

In addition to avoiding tap water with chemicals, one must also be careful of softened, distilled, reverse osmosis or other overly filtered water. These systems remove too many of the minerals. In turn, this water will leach minerals from your body and possibly leave you in a depleted condition. If you drink (or cook with) water softened with salt it is like a big salt shaker. Drinking living water hydrates cells and improves health. Drinking overly filtered water can actually dehydrate cells. There is debate as to the health benefits and risks of drinking filtered water.

Use tampons and sanitary napkins made of organic cotton without chlorine. The FDA detected dioxins and dozens of other substances in conventional tampons. Look for ones that contain no chlorine, fragrance, wax, surfactants or rayon.

Purchase non-bleached coffee filters. Napkins, toilet tissue and tampons should be purchased with caution. The EPA has determined that using bleached coffee filters alone can result in a lifetime exposure to dioxin that exceeds acceptable risks

Estrogen dominance is when your body has excess estrogen or estrogen like compounds in relation to the amount of progesterone. This almost always occurs when women have used birth control and are exposed to exogenous sources of "estrogen like" chemicals known as xenohormones. Estrogen dominance can be reduced by reducing your exposure to environmental xenoestrogens or other known xenohormones. Recent studies indicate that **bioidentical** progesterone cream helps to correct hormonal imbalances caused by exposure to xenoestrogens by balancing the excess estrogen.

Milk Thistle

Beyond the treatment of liver disorders, everyday care of the liver lays a cornerstone for health. Holistic doctors, who look beneath the symptoms of an illness to its underlying cause, often discover that the liver has had a role to play. This is true across a vast range of different ailments including exposure to endocrine disruptors. The herb commonly called milk thistle cleanses the body of xenoestrogens by strengthening the liver which becomes weakened and less able to function optimally from all pharmaceutical and chemical exposure. Whether a drug is prescribed or over the counter they all hamper the livers ability to keep you balanced hormonally.

Adapted by author from <http://www.womenlivingnaturally.com/articlepage.php?id=73> Dec 2013

Part I: Xenohormones And Your Health

Unseen, Unknown And damaging. We Can No Longer Afford To Ignore The Effects.

by John R. Lee, M.D. and Virginia Hopkins

I am frequently asked why postmenopausal women need progesterone. After all, a woman's progesterone levels naturally fall to close to zero after menopause.

My answer is that if women ate a perfect diet, got plenty of exercise, fresh air and sunshine, had no chronic stress, got plenty of sleep, and lived in a world free of environmental estrogens, there would normally be no need for progesterone after menopause. The reality is that virtually all of us eat too much sugar and processed flour, lack enough exercise, fresh air or sunshine, are chronically stressed, sleep deprived and are awash in a sea of environmental estrogens created from our modern technological world of plastics and pesticides.

While you can do something about changing your diet, sleep, exercise and stress, you may be unaware of how to avoid environmental estrogens, and that's what I want to address this month. (If you do have questions about diet, exercise and stress management, you'll find detailed information in my two *What Your Doctor May Not Know... books.*)

Why Xenohormones Threaten Our Very Existence As A Species

Women have also asked me why, if a woman's estrogen levels have dropped after menopause, environmental estrogens would harm them. Environmental estrogens can have unpredictable and damaging effects on your body because they behave differently from your own estrogens. They can also do severe damage to a developing fetus. I believe that environmental estrogens are the leading cause of the rising rate of prostate cancer in men, and that they play a significant role in the epidemic of infertility and PMS among young women.

Many of these chemicals can also damage the nervous system and the brain, contribute to the development of cancer, and cause birth defects. A study published in the *New England Journal of Medicine* in 1996 (J.L. Jacobson, et al) showed that mothers with the highest levels of the industrial toxins PCBs in their bodies had children who, by age 11, were three times more likely to have low IQ scores and to be at least two years behind in reading comprehension.

A very recent study published in the March issue of the *Journal of the American Medical Association* (JAMA) reported that women who were exposed to solvents in the workplace and had symptoms of solvent exposure while they were pregnant, had a 13-fold higher risk of giving birth to a baby with serious birth defects.

Take A Lesson From Birds And Alligators

Xenohormones, also called endocrine disruptors, are a large class of exogenous (originating outside the body) compounds. Our primary problem with them is that they damage developing tissues in the endocrine system, which includes the thyroid, the adrenal glands, the pituitary gland, the testicles and ovaries, and the pancreas (which produces insulin).

A damaged endocrine system can, in turn, damage the reproductive organs such as the prostate and uterus, the immune system, blood sugar balance, and the ability of the brain to communicate with these systems. While many xenohormones have estrogenic effects, they can also be anti-estrogenic in the sense that they bind to estrogen receptors and in effect block their own potential estrogenic effect.

Damage from xenohormone exposure varies depending on the dose, individuality, and the age at which the exposure occurred. Fully matured tissues are less sensitive to xenohormone exposure than immature tissues. Developing tissues, during the early stage of embryo life are extremely sensitive to xenohormone exposure. Exposure doses that would leave an adult unharmed may cause irreparable damage to a developing baby. The observable effects of this damage maybe imperceptible until adulthood. All animal studies show that prenatal (in the womb) and young offspring are at greater risk than adults.

At about day 18 to 23 days after conception, the baby's gonads are developing. If the baby exposed to xenohormones is male, the Sertoli cells in the testes are damaged and, when he grows up to adulthood, his sperm count is less than it should be. The average sperm count of men in industrialized countries has been steadily decreasing. One study found an average count of 100 million in 1950, 75 million in 1970 and 50 million in 1990. Many studies are even more disturbing. A man is considered sterile if his sperm count is below 20 million. If the baby is female, the follicle cells in her ovaries are damaged and, when she grows up to adulthood, many of the follicles are dysfunctional, leading to either failed ovulation or to lack of progesterone production. In that case, she becomes estrogen dominant and prone to early miscarriage.

Where Do Xenohormones Come From?

The vast majority of these xenohormones are man-made petrochemical products used in pesticides, cleaning agents, solvents, adhesives, emulsifiers, plastics and many other chemicals used in manufacturing and industry. They are found in food from crops sprayed with pesticides, in the out-gassing of the materials we build our homes and offices with, in cosmetics, in coloring agents, in the various sprays we use to kill insects on our pets, in our homes and in the weed killers and fungicides we use on our lawns and gardens.

Our knowledge of the effects of xenohormones comes primarily from observing wildlife populations exposed to them through industrial pollution of waterways and agricultural spraying. No type of living creature has been immune from xenohormone effects, including birds, amphibians, reptiles, mammals, fish and shellfish. Humans are susceptible to xenohormones, and our environmental exposure to these agents is increasing. It is almost impossible to avoid them: they are a twentieth century plague.

Phytohormones Vs. Xenohormones

Strictly speaking, hormonal compounds from plants, called phytohormones or phytoestrogens, which are found in soy and some herbs for example, also fit the definition of xenohormones. Phytohormones, however, are considerably less toxic than synthetic xenohormones, since in most cases humans have evolved in the context of eating these plants and we have adapted to them, often to our benefit. In that sense, phytoestrogens are natural instead of foreign ("xeno") to us. In fact, the human body has the ability to bind the more toxic phytohormones to proteins that reduce their effects and make them easier to eliminate safely. The body is unable to do this with synthetic xenohormones.

Even The Government Is Taking Action

The Environmental Protection Agency (EPA) is now mandated by Congress to test the toxicity of these suspect pollutants with the aim of removing the more toxic ones. This is a Herculean task since there are now at least 100,000 such environmental pollutants. The EPA has initiated a two-tier testing program in which the most toxic agents are first identified by rapid, automated laboratory tests. The first reports from these tests are beginning to trickle out, and the negative consequences of exposure to the suspect chemicals is clear.

How To Reduce Xenohormones Exposure

You can dramatically reduce your exposure to xenohormones by following some basic guidelines even though, at first glance, it may seem overwhelmingly difficult to avoid them.

The Guidelines

Assume that all pesticides, fungicides and herbicides are toxic and do whatever you can to avoid them. This means any pesticide or herbicide used to kill bugs, fungus or plants. Pregnant women should be especially careful and children are more susceptible than adults.

Avoid processed and packaged foods and eat primarily fresh, whole and preferably organic foods.

Store your food in glass containers and if you cover food with plastic wrap, never let it touch the food. Never microwave or heat food in a plastic container.

Invest in a good water filter rather than buying bottled water. (Please change the filter regularly or you will create other health problems.)

If you build a new home, do it without particle board, laminated wood, wood veneers or other materials that out-gas chemicals. Find carpets that are free of fumes and toxic adhesives.

Use detergents, soaps and shampoos that are "eco-friendly."

Avoid solvents. If you must use them, protect your skin (they enter the bloodstream quickly through the skin) and avoid breathing the fumes. There are solvents in nail polish and nail polish remover, which are very popular among young teens who are vulnerable to reproductive damage.

Keep soft plastic toys away from children, especially if they are at an age where everything is still going into their mouth.

This article was originally published in the John R. Lee, M.D. Medical Letter. Even though the letter is no longer published. many of the articles that appeared in it can be found on this website.

Adapted by author from <http://www.virginiahopkinstestkits.com/xenohormoneI.html>

Part II: Xenohormones In Your Environment

Rounding Up the Usual Suspects

When it comes to chemicals, assume the worst.

by John R. Lee, M.D. and Virginia Hopkins

While hundreds of thousands of chemicals on the market are virtually unstudied for their toxic effects, scientists have identified classes of compounds that present the most widespread exposures and the highest toxicity. Pesticides are by far the worst offenders, **but** the following xenohormones are worth avoiding whenever possible.

Phthalates: These are some of the most pervasive synthetic chemicals and are found in most plastics, inks, adhesives, vinyl flooring and some paints. For years they have been present in baby teething rings and children's toys. The highest exposure probably comes from the soft plastics our food is wrapped in, which leach phthalates directly into the food.

According to an EPA study published in the March issue of *Toxicology and Industrial Health*, when female rats were exposed to phthalates, their offspring showed a wide variety of abnormalities. Most striking were their effects as androgen (male hormone) blockers in male offspring, which included a reduction of testosterone levels, abnormalities in the male reproductive tract and testicular tumors among adult animals. Women exposed to high levels of phthalates have a higher risk of miscarriage. Most of Europe has already wisely phased out phthalates.

The same research group has also found that two fungicides (vinclozolin and procymidone), an herbicide (linuron), and an insecticide (methoxychlor) also cause reproductive abnormalities in rodents. Linuron caused male reproductive tract abnormalities that were hard to detect until autopsy and exposure to the herbicide just before puberty dramatically delayed the maturation of male sexual organs. The dosages at which these chemicals had their effects were close to the dosages at which humans are exposed.

Alkylphenols and nonylphenols: These xenohormones are found in detergents, shampoos, cosmetics, spermicidal lubricants, pesticides and clear plastics. They are washed into municipal sewage systems and are left intact during treatment, so they enter the food chain. In waterways that receive municipal water treatment runoff, highly concentrated amounts have been found in the flesh of fish and birds. Much of the tap water in the U.S. contains alkylphenolic compounds so you can be sure they are also accumulating in human flesh. These chemicals increase the growth rate of human breast cancer cells, and pregnant rats exposed to alkylphenol breakdown products had male offspring whose reproductive organs developed improperly. Much of Europe is already banning these substances.

Bisphenol A (BPA): The key component of polycarbonate resins, which are used in hard plastics. Those we are most exposed to include dental sealants primarily used on children's teeth, and the hard plastics used in food and drink containers and to coat the inside surfaces of water pipes and metal food packages. BPA has potent estrogenic effects in extremely small amounts, and seems to have an especially potent estrogenic effect on the prostate. The argument is over how much BPA is actually leached out by these plastics. Some researchers report finding no BPA in tests **but** a paper in the journal *Environmental Health Perspectives* by Nagal et al, found that "...the amount of bisphenol A required to cause significant prostate change is comparable, relative to body weight, of the amounts... found in saliva of children two years after the application of a polycarbonate dental sealant… and the amount recovered in the liquid portion within food cans lined by polycarbonate sealants."

Natural Alternatives To Pesticides

There are dozens of simple, practical and inexpensive ways to deter insects without pesticides. One of the most effective ways to protect both your outdoor plants, your vegetable garden and your home from most insects is a simple solution of Dr. Bronner's Pure-Castile Peppermint Soap and water: five drops of liquid soap to 1 quart of water. You can find the liquid Dr. Bronner's at your local health food store; a four to five dollar bottle could last years! This works for everything from ants to aphids to whiteflies.

Another simple solution for some of the tougher insects such as fleas, termites and cockroaches is boric acid, which is sold in tubs at most pet stores these days. It is benign to humans **but** very effectively kills these pests. It can be sprinkled at the edges of rooms where cockroaches are coming in, it can be dusted in carpets and furniture and then vacuumed up (enough will remain to kill insects for about a year) and it can be sprinkled under houses to kill termites.

This article was originally published in the John R. Lee, M.D. Medical Letter. Although the newsletter is no longer published, many of the articles that appeared in it can be found on this website.

Adapted by author from <http://www.virginiahopkinstestkits.com/xenohormoneII.html>

Ideal Nutrition

This is an ideal, that for now may beyond reach. You may want to try coming close to the ideal for a few days and adapt the parts that are doable and *feel* right for you.

NOTE	Avoid mixing the food together and avoid adding salt
NOTE	Eat with hands or wooden utensils
	Never combine starches with meats or sugars.
NOTE	Never eat pork, beef or animal organs. Eggs, milk, poultry and fish may be ok. Use your own guidance. Pine nuts and Sunflower seeds are suggested for protein sources.
NOTE	Eat beginning in the morning
NOTE	Eat fruits and vegetables that have been grown locally. Eat only vine-ripened produce. Eat vegetables raw or steamed.
Preparation	Acquire a small quantity of all the vegetables, fruits and edible herbs growing in the region where you live. Also acquire: honey, flower pollen, pine nut oil and spring water
Preparation	Go a whole day without eating. Drink only spring water and have a glass of red beet juice for lunch. (After drinking the beet juice it is better stay home.)
First Day	Upon awakening the following morning and *feeling* hungry, take any vegetable, herb or piece of fruit and put it on a small plate. After sitting down at the table, carefully observe what is lying on the plate; sniff it, lick it and then eat it with an unhurried chewing.
First Day	If still hungry or the next time you get hungry select a second piece (same item or something different)and eat it in the same manner as the first.
First Day	Take all the produce you have obtained and sample them in any sequence at short intervals as above. The sensation of hunger determines the time for sampling.
First Day	By the end of this day you should have sampled all locally grown produce. (If there is a large variety available and one day is insufficient, the sampling can extend to the following day.)

Second and Third Day	Cut each type of produce into small pieces and lay them out on a large plate. Any produce that will quickly spoil on the plate should be immersed in spring water. Remember the honey, flower pollen, pine nut oil and spring water
Second and Third Day	Go about your daily affairs. When you are hungry go over to the table and pick up an item you like and eat it. It is possible some of the food may be eaten up completely, while the rest may be left untouched. This means that your body selected for you what you needed at that moment, while what was unneeded was left untouched.
From Fourth Day On	Cut each type of produce that you have been eating into small pieces and lay them out on a large plate each morning Any produce that will quickly spoil on the plate should be immersed in spring water. Go about your daily affairs. When you are hungry go over to the table and pick up an item you like and eat it. There is no need to put uneaten produce on the table every day. Every fourth day a complete variety should once again be displayed. Your body may need something different by then. If you find that there is something consistently left uneaten, after a couple weeks you may want to skip buying it for a while and try it again later.
Away from Home	Put a portion of the food from the table into a cooler or basket. During the day, when you are hungry, pick an item you like from the basket and eat it. Anastasia recommends a small birch-bark container.
Extended Trip	Become familiar with the produce available in the new territory, since, in spite of identical names, there may be significant taste and nutritional differences. See First Day, Second and Third Day and From Fourth Day On

Above table created by author based largely on Vladimir Megre, Book # 8.1: *The New Civilization,* pages 63-66 of The Ringing Cedars Series and partly on Mary Summer Rain, *Earhtway,* pages 46 - 54

Chapter 2

Daily Practices

Upgrade Internal Dialog And Verbal Communication

Realize that all thoughts as well as words are dialogue. If you have a thought of, "I'm ugly" or "They are crazy" the thought carries almost as much negative energy or judgment as saying it out load. Watch your thoughts as well as your words. You can always say to yourself silently or out load if appropriate, "Cancel/Clear", and think of a positive.

There are many ways to practice this. The main key is to be aware of your thoughts and words and practice keeping them positive and Loving to the best of your ability.

Words To Avoid Using

List: *not, n't* as in *don't and can't, hate, try, should, would, could, need to, stop* as in "stop it"

The Word *Not*

Be positive and avoid the word *not* (includes *n't*)

The Universe only understands 'yes'. It is critical to use the positive counterpart of any negative. If you say, "I will not be Angry" or "I am not angry", the Universe hears, "I will be angry" or "I am angry". Instead say, "I will be forgiving, LOVING" or "I am forgiving, LOVING" (unconditional love). If you have difficulty thinking of an appropriate word, use the positive word or words that come the closest.

Interestingly, when you think or say, "I am not happy", the universe keeps the 'not' in place and energizes the opposite of happy.

With The Word *not*	Reworded to Avoid the word *not*
Not interesting	Boring
Not honest	Dishonest
Not important	Trifling/Unimportant
Not paying attention	Ignoring
Not big	Small
Not known	Unknown
I'm not angry	I am Loving
I'm not judgmental	I am in a state of unconditional acceptance
I'm not Happy	I am happy.
Don't touch the stove. It's hot. (don't = do not)	The stove is hot. Stay away from the burners.
Don't run in the house	Walk in the house, please

The Word *but*

The word *but* negates what was said before the *but*. Use a period and new sentence, the word *and* or the word *however*.

The word *Hate*

May be the most damaging word to the Spirit. Definitely diametrically opposed to LOVE. Do your absolute best to avoid using this word. Enough said.

The word *Try*

If you are 'trying' you are keeping whatever you are trying to do in the future instead of 'doing'. You may also be implying failure.

With The Word *try*	Reworded to Avoid the word *try*
"I'm trying to do by best."	" I am doing my best."
"I'm trying to tie my shoe."	"I am learning to tie my shoe."
I'm trying to get a garden going."	"I am starting a garden."
" I try to be loving."	"I am loving to the best of my ability."

The Word *Should*

Trying to reduce stress and telling yourself that you *should* , only creates more stress.

Let go of what you think others expect of you. If you try to meet others people's expectations you may beat yourself up with a bunch of *shoulds* that come from other peoples values instead of your own.

Too often we attempt to impose our will on other people by telling them what they 'SHOULD' do. What we are really saying is, 'our way is the right way, it is the only one way'. Are you trying to be helpful with your suggestions or is your ego leading the way? Use alternative phrases such as "Have you considered doing it like this?" or "This way worked for me".

The Word *Should* and the 'Inner Critic'

Should is one of the favorite words of the formidable inner critic. In this case, *shoulds* may come from your inner critic's tendency to find fault with you no matter what, instead of from your heartfelt values. **Even perfection will be judged lacking by the inner critic**. An active inner critic will hit you with a barrage of *shoulds* and *should nots* for the sole purpose of making you *feel* bad. This is what inner critics do.

The Word *Could*

The Word *Would*

The Word *Need*

Sometimes use of the word need is ok, as in "I need a new pair of shoes" if your shoes are worn out or outgrown. If you have shoes you are bored of, it becomes a want rather than a need. We actually need very few things to live comfortably on earth.

The Word *Stop* (as in "stop it")

Punctuation

Example of Importance: "Execute never, show mercy." or "Execute, never show mercy."

Speaking, Communicating And Doing Your Best

Words lacking LOVE are simply misuse of "The Word". This can put negative, limiting and damaging thoughts and beliefs in another's mind. This can be an unaware use of the word with no ill intent.

A sensitive person can be affected by thoughts without verbalization and therefore needs to be aware that when he or she senses the thoughts of others they can be de-energized without taking them on. Think of them as un-verbalized words.

Speak Truth With LOVE

Speak with integrity. Say only what you mean. Avoid speaking against yourself or others. If you are exhausted, have a headache, or just *feel* ill, do your best to ask the other person or group to allow you what you need.

What will really make a difference is practice and action.

Allow Others Their Projections

Remember that other peoples' reactions towards you are their projections coming from their choices and perception.

If someone gives you an opinion or says unkind or judgmental words, realize that this person is dealing with his or her own *feelings*, beliefs, and opinions. If you notice your own mind being judgmental and critical, realize it is a part of you that is asking for healing.

Learn to recognize words, thoughts and actions as Love or Something Else by practicing *feeling* and *awareness*. This will help you to trust yourself more and become more LOVING.

As you make a habit of taking nothing personally, there is no need to place your trust in what others say or do or to defend yourself from others' words or thoughts. When you truly understand this, and no longer take things personally, the careless comments or actions of others will be unable to hurt you.

What will really make a difference is practice and action.

Clear Communication

With clear communication, all of your relationships will change for the better

Find the courage to ask questions and to express what you really want. Communicate with others as clearly as you can without making assumptions. Avoid misunderstandings. Ask what the other person or group wants and let them know what you want.

What will really make a difference is practice and action.

Always Do Your Best

Always do your best, being aware that your best varies moment to moment. By doing your best there is no perceived need for self judgment. Unconditionally accept yourself.

What will really make a difference is practice and action.

Be careful to avoid, "I am doing my best", as an excuse.

Personal Notes

_____
_____
_____
_____
_____
_____
_____
_____
_____
_____
_____
_____

Chapter 3

What Is Man?

A constriction of overall human thought has been reflected in a narrowing of the meaning of *man*, which originally - like Russian *chelovek* and German *Mensch* designated all humanity, both men and women, as *thinking, intelligent beings* This constriction began around the eleventh century A.D. in various languages

This is an opportunity to rediscover the *original meaning* of a word whose usage has been constricted and corrupted over the past ten centuries.

Hence it was decided to translate *chelovek,* wherever appropriate to the context, to the term *Man* with a capital M in an effort to retain the association of the term with a divine (as opposed to a material, earthly) origin and to draw upon the original, uncorrupted meaning of the word *man* as a manifestation of ' eternal Mind' - implied in the etymology of the Russian term *chelovek.* So let *all* readers of this book be put on notice: whenever you see *Man* with a capital M, this includes *you.*

Human (as in human being):

This term has the problem in that it suggests a formation of the species from matter, or earth.

Humus - the organic constituent of soil is associated with lowly concepts, such as *humble* and *humility.* Also, the word *human* is essentially an adjective even though commonly used as a noun in today's English. *

* Vladimir Megre, Translators Preface, Book # 1: *Anastasia,* of The Ringing Cedars Series

For those that believe we were made in Gods' Image, I suggest the image is Man as in "*thinking, intelligent being*". Men and women as in "human being" are energized by Mans Spirit.

I like to think of myself as "Man" (*thinking, intelligent being and spirit*), then "human being" and then "man".

"I am Man. I am a human being. I am a man".

If you are a woman you may think of yourself as "Man" (*thinking, intelligent being and spirit*), then "human being" and then "woman".

"I am Man. I am a human being. I am a woman".

Personal Notes

_____
_____
_____
_____
_____
_____
_____
_____
_____
_____
_____

Chapter 4

Balance And The Nature Of Duality

Yin Yang symbol, also known as also known as the Tai Chi symbol

The image consists of a circle divided into two teardrop-shaped halves - one white and the other black. Within each half is contained a smaller circle of the opposite color.

In terms of Taoist cosmology, the circle represents the Tao - the undifferentiated Unity out of which all of existence arises. The black and white halves within the circle represent Yin-qi and Yang-qi - the primordial feminine and masculine energies whose interplay gives birth to the manifest world.

Smaller Circles Within The Larger Circle:

What's great about the Yin-Yang symbol is that the smaller circles nested within each half of the symbol serve as a constant reminder of the interdependent nature of the black/white "opposites." It reminds the Taoist practitioner that all of relative existence is in constant flux and change.

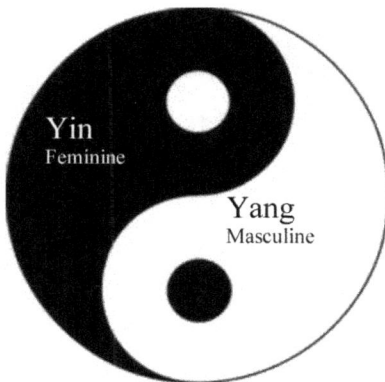

Yin Yang originates in ancient Chinese philosophy and metaphysics, which describes two primal opposing **but** complementary forces found in all things in the universe. Yin, the darker element, is passive, dark, feminine, downward-seeking, and corresponds to the night; yang, the brighter element, is active, light, masculine, upward-seeking and corresponds to the day. Yin is often symbolized by water, while yang is symbolized by fire. The theory is that all things in the universe have an opposing force, and though they are opposing, they are very interconnected.

It symbolizes the balancing of opposite forces and the dual nature of duality. There is a third element that is often left unmentioned. This third element is represented by the circle which represents Containment, The Whole, Finiteness. Without the containment the opposing elements could not exist, much less maintain their balance.

They are different, and distinct, yet one could **not** exist without the other. The circle itself - which contains these two halves - is like the metal (silver, gold or copper) of the coin. It is what the two sides have in common - what makes them "the same."

The yin yang symbol can be considered a symbol of balance within duality. What is outside the circle is beyond duality. It is also a symbol of universal harmony and balance.

What is outside the circle? Non-duality and Undifferentiated infinite energy.

Chapter 5

The Importance of the Subconscious and How to Strengthen Your Connection and Intuition

<u>There is nothing sub about the subconscious mind</u>.

The subconscious is more in touch with 'Reality' than the conscious mind.

It is vitally important to have a Loving, clear and cooperative relationship with your subconscious mind.

Thesaurus for 'sub': subordinate, secondary and junior, which are all adjectives.
     This DOES **NOT** describe the subconscious mind.

Thesaurus for 'conscious': aware, awake, cognizant which are all adjectives.
     The subconscious is more aware and awake than the conscious mind. Without the subconscious the conscious mind is pretty much asleep.

The super-conscious and conscious minds seem to be ok with being adjectives.

I prefer the Hawaiian name, Unihipili, for the subconscious mind. The Unihipili is more in touch with 'Reality' than the conscious mind. It may be lost and need guidance from the conscious mind to connect to LOVE, and once it is connected to LOVE it will help the conscious mind and all aspects of you connect more strongly to LOVE. If you consciously chose "Anything Else" the Unihipili will connect you to something other than LOVE.

I will be referring to the subconscious mind as Unihipili in most instances.

Willpower comes from the conscious mind. The cooperation of the Unihipili is needed for the choices to remain in effect.

The Unihipili (subconscious mind or child within) will respond or react according to your "choice." This child within is different than "the inner child" as used in inner child healing and soul retrieval. The inner child as used in 'inner child work' and soul retrieval **is a part of** the Unihipili.

As we increase the clarity and strength of communication between our conscious mind and the Unihipili, new energy, greater understanding, improved creativity and a knowingness of our life purpose will develop.

The Unihipili can also be thought of as the Gatekeeper. Some of our *feelings* and beliefs become our Gatekeeper. As you begin to become aware of and develop a LOVING relationship with the Unihipili (gatekeeper) your awareness of and access to the unknowable will also develop. Part of the Unihipili's purpose is to protect us from becoming overwhelmed by accessing too much all at once.

The Unihipili is the link between the conscious mind and the super-conscious mind. Without this link/interpreter there is no connection, or a very weak and unconscious link.

Conceptual Graphic Of Unihipili

The graphic below was created by the author.

Unihipili as Gatekeeper:

> The Unihipili allows access to information from other dimensions/realities to the extent you are ready. It keeps you from being overwhelmed. Your conscious mind and conscious choices determine whether it connects to Divine LOVE or Anything Else.

Unihipili as Interpreter:

> The realm of Spirit normally does **not** speak your native language (for me it is English). We normally grasp the meaning as a rapid flow of thoughts, images, memories, feelings, concepts and awareness. There is often very little time to think about what you are receiving, and if you stop to think and analyze the flow usually stops. Save the analyzing and thinking until after the flow stops.

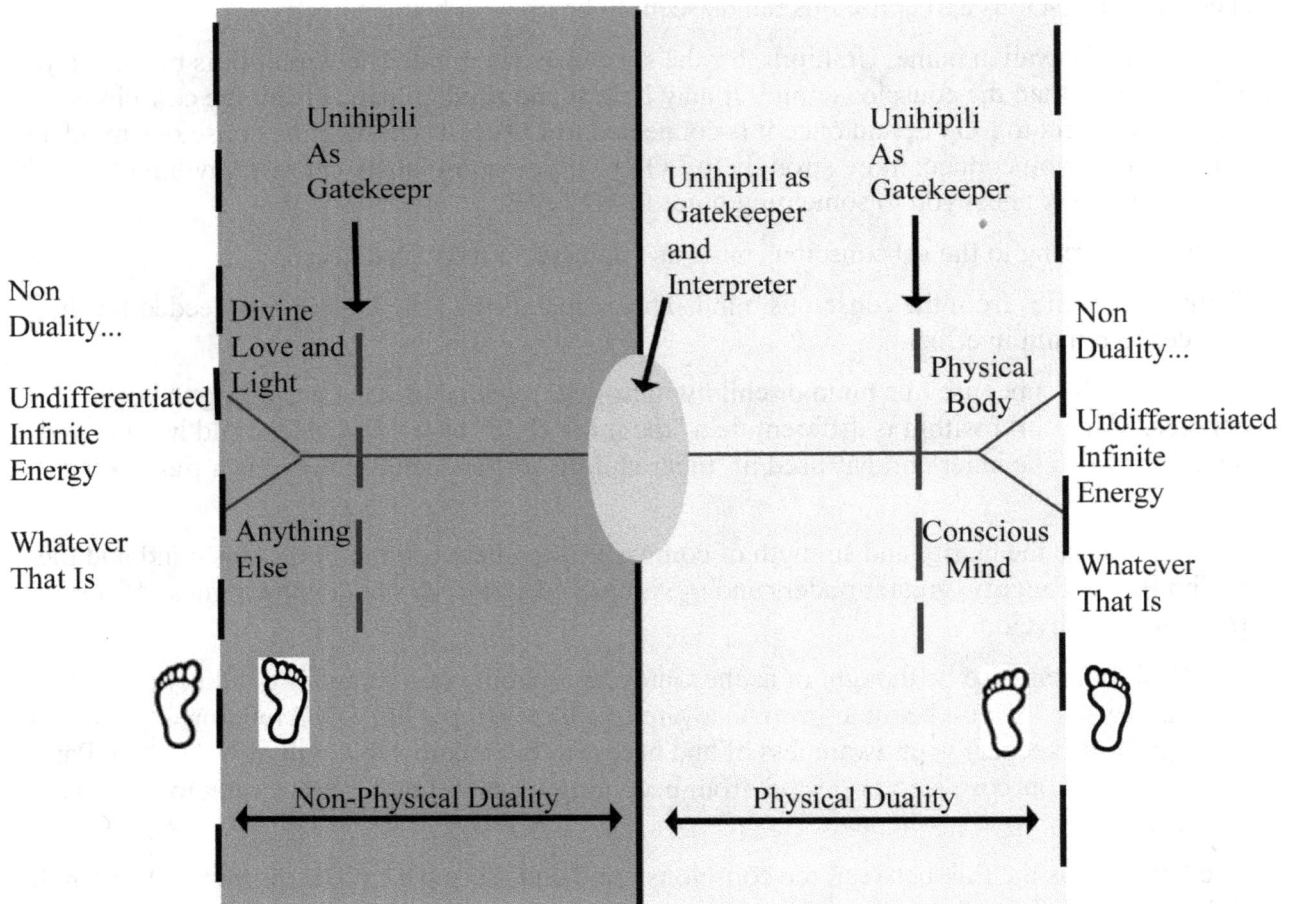

Unihipili
As
Gatekeepr

Unihipili as
Gatekeeper
and
Interpreter

Unihipili
As
Gatekeeper

Non
Duality...

Undifferentiated
Infinite
Energy

Whatever
That Is

Divine
Love and
Light

Anything
Else

Physical
Body

Conscious
Mind

Non
Duality...

Undifferentiated
Infinite
Energy

Whatever
That Is

Non-Physical Duality

Physical Duality

Another Conceptual Graphic Of Unihipili

The graphic below was created by the author.

I prefer the Hawaiian Name, Unihipili, for the subconscious mind

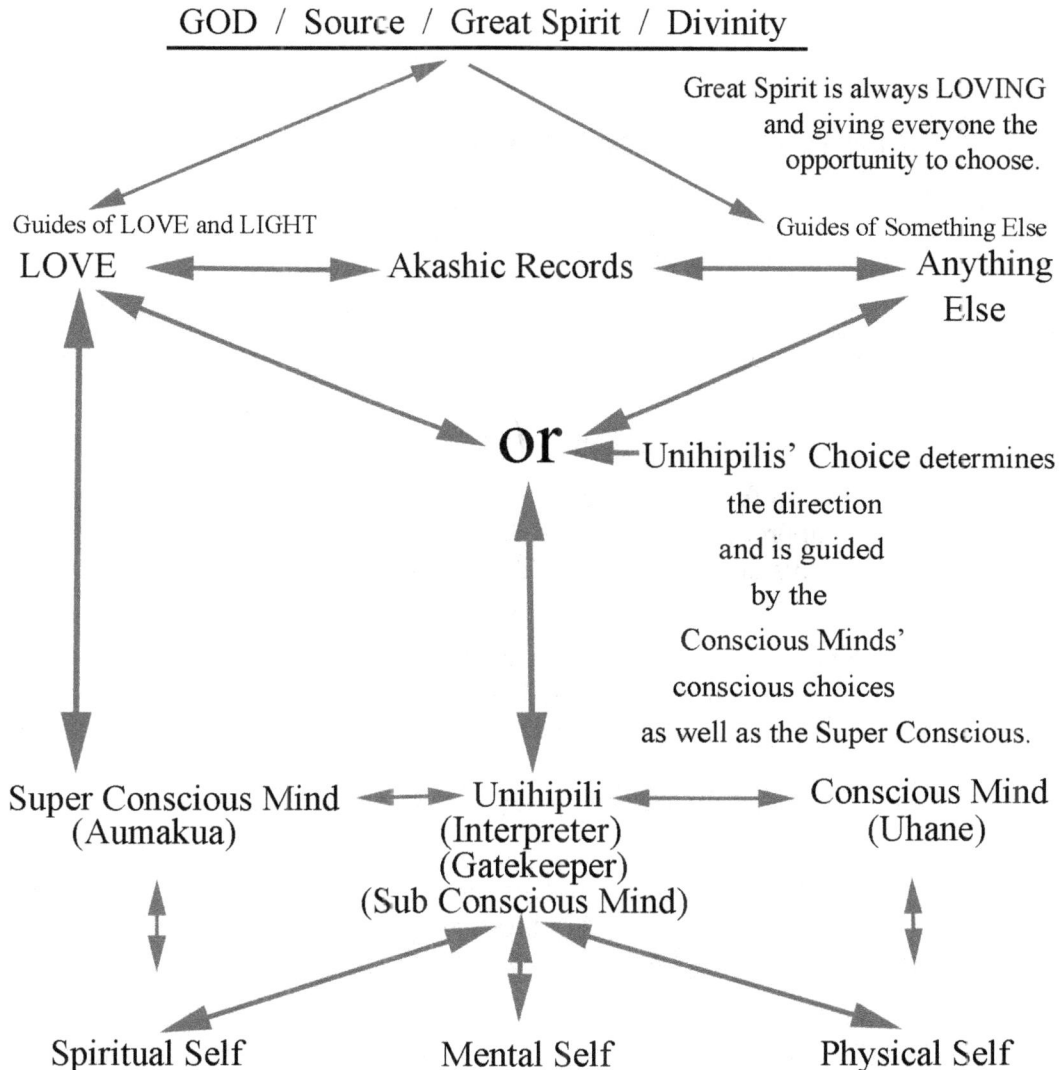

GOD / Source / Great Spirit / Divinity

Great Spirit is always LOVING and giving everyone the opportunity to choose.

Guides of LOVE and LIGHT
LOVE ⟷ Akashic Records ⟷ Anything Else
Guides of Something Else

or ← Unihipilis' Choice determines
the direction
and is guided
by the
Conscious Minds'
conscious choices
as well as the Super Conscious.

Super Conscious Mind ⟷ Unihipili ⟷ Conscious Mind
(Aumakua) (Interpreter) (Uhane)
(Gatekeeper)
(Sub Conscious Mind)

Spiritual Self   Mental Self   Physical Self

Willpower comes from the conscious mind. The cooperation of the Unihipili is needed for the choices to remain in effect.

Exercise To Connect To Your Unihipili With LOVE

To let the Unihipili know it is loved and to teach it and your conscious mind to communicate with each other and the Divine as is best, I suggest you do the following. This exercise will help you and your Unihipili's connection to become stronger and more loving.

Unihipili can be thought of as 'you' too. During the exercise the Unihipili will be referred to as *'U'*.

Exercise to consciously connect with your Unihipili:

From a state of LOVE, say hello to your Unihipili. "Hello, I love you and am happy that we are strengthening our bond. Please show me a representation of what you look like and/or give me a sense of you. *Thank you.*

You may get a vision and/or *feeling* of a very small child who is sad, lost, lonely and/or angry. Then again, you may find a happy child who is already fairly mature, connected, happy and LOVING.

Ask permission before continuing to strengthen the bond with LOVE using steps 1-4 below:

1) Hold your hands out in front of you, at shoulder level, with the palms up, in invitation. Allow the Unihipili to approach. When you see or sense that *'U'* is present and ready, position your hands, palms down, on Unihipili's shoulders with LOVE.
When it *feels* right, ask Unihipili, "Are we ready for the next exercise?"

2) Again hold your hands out in front of you, at shoulder level, with your palms down. Allow the Unihipili to approach you and stand up so your hands are touching the top of *'U's''* head. Gently stroke the top of *'U's''* head or just allow *'U'* to stand there and experience your LOVE.
When it *feels* right, ask Unihipili, "Are we ready for the next exercise?"

3) Now hold your arms out wide, with your palms facing in, and allow Unihipili to approach you. Allow *'U'* to hug you, and only when invited, slowly, gently and lovingly close your arms for a mutual hug. Allow Unihipili to experience your LOVE.
When it *feels* right, ask Unihipili, "Are we ready for the next exercise?"

4) Finally, hold your hands out in front of you at waist level with your palms up. Allow the Unihipili to approach you and put *'U's''* hand on yours. You may stroke each other's hands to share the LOVE.
When it *feels* right, tell Unihipili, "I love you and thank you". Be open to any response and when done open your eyes.

Only with reverence, LOVE, and self-discipline will you win your Unihipili's cooperation. When allowed, Unihipili will respond automatically and you will have a renewed and powerful helper.

Remember to maintain communication with your Unihipili and to support Unihipili, realizing that even though it is very powerful, 'U' is in many ways childlike and innocent.

Preferably every morning and evening, or at least when prompted, request the following:

1) "Unihipili, please always remember to stay connected to and accept things from Great Spirit and Great Spirit's Helpers of Pure Divine LOVE and LIGHT only."

2) "Is there anything you want or need: toys, nourishment, clothes, swim/bath/shower, laundry bag, backpack, laundry done or guidance by me or Great Spirit"? Allow the Unihipili to choose as long as what 'U' chooses is of Pure Divine LOVE and LIGHT.

Remember the Unihipili is present in a non-physical realm, so 'U' is free from the rules of the physical world. The Unihipili can wear anything 'U' wants; eat as much as 'U' wants; have 'U's" backpack as large or as small as 'U' wants, and any color. The backpack and its contents are also free from the rules of the physical world and can be expanded or contracted as the Unihipili desires, therefore the Unihipili can carry as much as 'U' wants by shrinking and then re-expanding the items. Allow "U" to play!

Personal Notes

_____

_____

_____

_____

_____

_____

_____

_____

_____

_____

_____

_____

_____

_____

Chapter 6
Channels, Mediums And Clarity

Dictionary Definitions Of Channel, Channeling and Flow

<u>channel</u>:

    canal, conduit, straight, control, focus, direct, concentrate

<u>channeling</u>:

    The act or practice of serving as a medium through which a spirit guide purportedly communicates with living persons. The esoteric process of receiving messages or inspiration from extra-dimensional beings or spirits, whereby one is a medium or channel for such an entity. In physics, the process that constrains the path...

<u>flow</u>:

    run, pour, flood, stream, gush, surge, spring, arise, emerge, emanate, issue, well up. Flow is the mental state of operation in which a person performing an activity is fully immersed in energized focus and full involvement in the process of the activity. In essence, flow is characterized by complete absorption in what one does.

Flow Proposed By Mihaly Csikszentmihaly

Csikszentmihalyi is noted for his work in the study of happiness and creativity, **but** is best known as the architect of the notion of *flow* and for his years of research and writing on the topic. He is the author of many books and over 120 articles or book chapters. Martin Seligman, former president of the American Psychological Association, described Csikszentmihalyi as the world's leading researcher on positive psychology. This positive psychological concept has been widely referenced across a variety of fields.

According to Csikszentmihalyi, flow is completely focused motivation. It is a single-minded immersion and represents perhaps the ultimate experience in harnessing the emotions in the service of performing and learning. In flow, the emotions are more than just contained and channeled; they are positive, energized, and aligned with the task at hand. To be caught in the ennui (a *feeling* of utter weariness, listlessness, discontent/ dissatisfaction, lack of interest, boredom) of depression or the agitation of anxiety is to be barred from flow. The hallmark of flow is a *feeling* of spontaneous joy, even rapture while performing a task. Flow is also described as a deep focus on nothing except the activity - even oneself or one's emotions are put aside.

Flow has many of the same characteristics as the positive aspects of hyper-focus. However, hyper-focus is sometimes described in less glowing terms. For examples, some cases of spending "too much" time playing video games, or of getting side-tracked and pleasurably absorbed by one aspect of an assignment or task to the detriment of the assignment in general. In some cases, hyper-focus can "grab" a person, perhaps causing him to appear unfocused or to start several projects and complete few. Colloquial terms for this or similar mental states include: to be in the moment, present, in the zone, on a roll, wired in, in the groove, on fire, in tune, centered, or singularly focused. * *
<http://en.wikipedia.org/wiki/Mihaly_Csikszentmihalyi> January 2014

Receiving Your Own Guidance

Even the information from an intermediary with good intentions can be distorted by their beliefs, habits and ideas. When you are nervous or upset you will receive either distorted information or none at all. Calm yourself and invite only intermediaries which are positive and LOVING. Use your own intuition as to the accuracy of the information. As you continue to receive information your capacity to receive increases. Never color the impressions with your own personal ideas. Step aside and receive the messages quickly without deliberation or thought no matter how silly they seem. Do your analyzing after the thought stream is over.

We all have access to the whole Universe - both visible and invisible. Every Man (man and woman) may communicate with anything or anyone. It works pretty much the same as through your radio receiver.

There are so many stations broadcasting all kinds of information, out of which the owner of the receiver must select (choose) what he is going to listen to.

Man is both the receiver and its owner. And which source finds a reception in his thought depends on his conscious awareness, his *feelings* and purity. As a rule, a Man receives information he is able to make sense of, understand and use. All this must take place calmly and quietly, without intrusive attention drawn to greatness.

What Is Distortion? How Is It Recognized?

When voices draw attention to their own greatness, they try to appeal to one's sense of self-importance: "Look here, I'm so great, yet I have chosen only you out of everyone - you shall be my pupil, and you too shall be greater than everyone else." As a rule, this is what you would hear from Beings of something other than LOVE and LIGHT. They act on Man's mind, his sense of self-importance and his fear of the unknown.

Every Man produces their own thoughts and everyone's thoughts still exist. They always remain in what some call the Akashic records without disappearing into oblivion.

Only one's own purity is capable of hearing Truth undistorted. There are a multitude of sources, all of them claiming to be Truth. You are free to listen to them or to tune them out.

Adapted by author from Vladimir Megre, Book # 3: *The Space of Love,* pages 187-191 of The Ringing Cedars Series

You are free to decide; to choose. Listen to LOVE or Anything Else.

Knowing When The Source Is Communicating Truth

When Truth Is Being Perceived Without Interference

When Truth is being perceived without interference you hear more than just words. Suddenly there is a flash of a LOVING *feeling* or emotion in the soul, accompanied by sensations of warmth and peace.

When the source of information is from other than LOVE or there is interference, it often comes as an order or command. Even if it is disguised as a request it will *feel* less than LOVING. It may even talk about love and good. It may seem wise, even very wise. The originating source often claims to be supreme and very powerful. Know this: it is of something other than LOVE and is hiding behind good.

Adapted by author from Vladimir Megre, Book # 3: *The Space of Love,* pages 187-191 of The Ringing Cedars Series

Prophecy

Have your own connection to Great Spirit and LOVE for intuition, awareness and knowing. Any other source is incomplete or distorted and questionable. Listen to your-self before listening to anyone else.

Prophecy, as normally defined, is a process in which one or more messages that have been communicated to a prophet are then communicated to others. Such messages typically involve divine inspiration, interpretation, or revelation of conditioned events to come. The process of prophecy especially involves reciprocal communication of the prophet with the divine source of the messages.

The dates of the fearful cataclysms upon the Earth were the creations of thought even though some think they are divinations. These thoughts, passed off as prophecies, made millions of people believe in gloom and doom and then their thoughts energized implementation of the same. These thoughts still hover up there, hiding in the blue, still frightening people and need LOVE to be de-energized.

Many teachers, gurus, sages, and prophets try to suggest to Man that he is abject and weak in spirit, knows nothing of himself and that all Truths are accessible only to a few select like themselves. They teach that you can detect LOVE'S voice and the Truth only through them. Many foretell gloom for Man, thereby creating both gloom and hell with their thoughts and the thoughts of those who listen to them.

Let go of the of dogma, conventions and fear. LOVE instead, thereby creating a place of LOVE.

Adapted by author from Vladimir Megre, Book # 3: *The Space of Love,* pages 227 - 228 of The Ringing Cedars Series

Subjugation

Be your own guide. No book, including sacred texts, or guru or teacher can be a complete and accurate map for *your* path. Until you have made 'the journey' yourself how to you know which ones are right. Follow your own feeling, intuition and guidance above all others.

Recent philosophical concepts gave rise to religion like philosophical tendencies. A dominant concept in our lifetime has turned out to be the concept of subjugation to some kind of Supreme Mind. Its precise location is unimportant, be it in the infinite spaces of the "All That Is" or localized in the essence of a particular human soul. Much more important is the fact that the concept of subjugation dominates over everything else if allowed. After that come the particulars - subjugation to a teacher, a mentor or a ritual.

No one who subjugates themselves can be truly happy. No single person on the Earth can be fully happy as long as such a concept is dominant in Man's consciousness.

The Universe itself is a thought, a thought which is partially visible as matter. When you approach the edge of all creation, your thought will reveal a new beginning and continuation.

Most, maybe all, predictions of fearful cataclysms on the Earth, were created by someone's own thought which persuaded people to accept their implementation through fear. These thoughts are still hovering over the Earth, still frightening people with their sense of despair. The more people believe in universal doom the greater the image, thereby increasing the possibility it will come to pass. The more people believe in and practice LOVE, the more positive and loving the future.

Adapted by author from Vladimir Megre, Book # 4: *Co-Creation,* page 41 and Book # 5: *Who Are We?*, pages 157 - 163 of The Ringing Cedars Series

Let go of fear and others' thoughts of gloom and doom and instead embrace LOVE and LIGHT. If enough people practice LOVE and let go of fear, the gloom and doom will no longer come true.

Chapter 7
Knowing, *Feeling*, Awareness And Judgment
What Is "Knowing"? And What Is
"Being Fully Aware"?

There is a difference between "knowing" (*znat'*) and "being fully aware of" *(vedat)* something.

Znat' is "knowing" in Russian and *Vedat* is "being fully aware of" in Russian. Notice that they are single words. As far as I know there is no single word in English that denotes "being fully aware of".

"Being fully aware of" is more than to just "know". It is to *feel* with one's whole being - body and soul - a multitude of phenomena, the purpose of each Divine creation, as well as His system.

And every Man was once fully aware that what he consumed as food filled the soul with conscious awareness, as well as feeding the body.

The words *znat'* and *vedat'* in Russian are often used interchangeably in the sense of "know", whereas in fact there is a significant distinction between them. *Znat'* specifically refers to "knowing" through the mind or logic. V*edat'* (from an ancient Sanskrit root) covers other kinds of knowing as well - inspiration, intuition, emotional *feelings* etc.) - in other words, more than just "knowing" per se. V*edat'* is being fully aware of all dimensions of a subject through all the various means of communicating knowledge.

Thinking and using the logical, knowing, mind is fine, however avoid wallowing in all your information and contemplations. Also, *feel* this information.

The answers to all questions are right here in space, right with us. We only need to know how to perceive them and make them manifest. The answer "lives" in you.

Decide what's real by yourself; with your "self". You will, with practice, be able to *feel* both matter and what is invisible in equal measure.

We tend to go digging around in all that information in the mind, trying to define it with our mind. You need more than your mind to get it. The mind is unable to fathom the volume of information known and available to each individual.

Feel with your "self", all planes of being.

You need to *feel* the spiritual and the material in equal measure. When one predominates over the other, it's like a person going lame. When *feeling* the spiritual and the material in equal measure you'll be able to take a solid stand in life, with both feet planted firmly on the ground and with a clear connection to Great Spirit.

Adapted by author from Vladimir Megre, Book # 6: *The Book Of Kin,* page 144 and Book # 4: *Co-Creation,* page 229 of The Ringing Cedars Series

Difference Between

Awareness, Knowing And Judgment

Dictionary definitions

Awareness:
knowing something; noticing or realizing something

Knowing:
having knowledge, information or understanding

Judgment:
verdict, finding, sentence, opinion, belief, assessment

How I define them:

Awareness:
inspiration, intuition, *feelings*. Being fully aware of all dimensions of a subject through all the various means of communicating knowledge with LOVE.

Knowing:
knowing through the logical mind or logic.

Judgment:
Finding someone or something to be lacking or of inferior quality based on your opinions and beliefs. Finding someone or something to be superior or better based on your opinions and beliefs.

How To Recognize When You Are Sliding From Awareness Into Judgment

With awareness there is no *thought* of right or wrong, good or bad, Light or Dark, LOVE or Un-love. There is no *feeling* of being superior or inferior in any way. With awareness there is no need to defend yourself from others opinion, beliefs or words and no reason to try to justify yourself. There is also no inclination or attempt to "fix" them.

If you tag, name or label something or someone as good, bad, better than, worse than, superior or inferior, it is a judgment. Allow it to be an *awareness with feeling* that something or someone is out of harmony with you.

If I *feel* uncomfortable around someone or am in a place and *feel* that it is best that I disengage, I do my best to disengage lovingly. I quite often am unaware as to why. It's simply out of harmony with me. I just follow my *feeling* and guidance.

If something *feels* right and LOVING I do my best to make sure I am connected to "Great Spirit and Great Spirit Helpers as are best" and stay engaged as long as it is for the highest good.

Occasionally I *feel* something is off and at the same time *feel* it is best to share. I maintain extra diligence and vigilance as long as I am engaged. I disengage as soon as I am guided to.

Wisdom and Power

Power As In Glossary

Power - Dictionary Definition:

Authority, control, influence, supremacy, command, dominance, force.

Manipulation would be the key word; the power to manipulate situations and those around you.

Power - As Used In This Book:

Personal power comes from wisdom. Real personal power is a subtle quality of Beingness rather than a force.

Real power has nothing to do with control, especially the control of others. Conversely, real power is surrendering to the highest good.

Real power naturally settles within one's Beingness of its own accord as Wisdom and Love increase.

Wisdom As In Glossary

Wisdom - Dictionary Definition:

Understanding, knowledge, intelligence, accumulated learning, opinion widely held, accumulated philosophic or scientific learning, the judicious application of knowledge.

Wisdom - As Used In This Book

Wisdom has nothing to do with the level of one's attained knowledge, age, intelligence or I.Q. rating. Wisdom is born of LOVE arising from the heart. Wisdom becomes part of your Being.

Some aspects of wisdom: Acceptance, Patience and Perseverance, Attitude, Silence, Personal Responsibility, Gentleness and Serenity, Value and Priorities, and Respect.

True Wisdom is beyond words and the intellect, and is only fully understood by the heart through Awareness.

Wisdom Expanded

To understand wisdom as clearly as possible with the intellect, the main aspects of wisdom also need to be understood.

Acceptance:

Acceptance precludes judgment. It instills one's power to gracefully accept the "bad" behavior of others without inciting negativity within self. This has nothing to do with apathy. Acceptance is also letting go. It's releasing the compelling urge to understand another's behavior. Understanding, as a part of acceptance, impels us to make alternate choices and plans when life presents "misfortunes" or paths that somehow seem to go awry. Release the compelling urge to understand the *precise* reasons for another's behavior. Trying to find precise reasons is usually unimportant - and may only hold you back. Acceptance is the impetus that soothingly eases one forward into a gentle state where healing begins to take hold. Even when accepting the behavior of others, your emotional responses are still intact; you can still be hurt, disappointed, or saddened. Yet having acceptance is the singular quality that eases the personal harm that could have been inflicted. After a time, acceptance becomes easier and easier to do until it's an automatic responsive attitude.

Obviously, you still protect yourself as needed.

Patience and Perseverance:

When an outcome is imminent, as in waiting to have a child born, the element of anticipation accompanies the waiting period and that aspect serves to intensify and sweeten the manifested event. It's the long-term waiting that is destructive by stealing away the present. Patience and perseverance give the power to have goals without allowing those same goals to overshadow and darken daily living. Goals are of the future and, having the wisdom to realize that perspective gives one power to live every day to the fullest with patience, while holding on to those goals with perseverance. This prevents inner tension and turmoil, bringing a good measure of serenity to one's life.

Silence:

Knowing when to hold your tongue and your thoughts is wise. What's left unsaid can have a huge impact. There are situations when one's silence speaks louder than words. Silence is wise when it circumvents inflicting emotional pain or forcing your beliefs on others. This type of silence refers to guarding one's speech and even ones thoughts. Silence can be a gentle expression of kindness. A lot of talk is done to get attention or sympathy or make a bid for some type of control, which exposes a lack of wisdom.

Refraining from giving people answers to certain questions is wise. This lack of response is wise when a person, for one reason or another, refuses to take personal responsibility for their life; when they refuse to make their own decisions. Giving out answers to another's life questions steals away that individual's power to work through problems. It steals away their power to reason things out on their own. It steals away their beautiful gift of free will. It reeks of control.

Is there a need to defend oneself against falsehoods?

Personal Responsibility:

In regards to behavioral choices and decision making, when asking advice from friends, family, associates or psychics and trusting them above one's-self, folks are admitting that they are unable to control their lives, are unwilling to make a decision or take responsibility of a decision, and want someone else to tell them what to do. This gives power to others to control their lives. They let themselves become manipulated. They offer others power over them on a polished, silver platter.

It's wise to realize that your life is yours alone. Only you end up answering for how your life was enacted. It's having power when one understands that the absolute administration of their own life is their responsibility.

Remember, this is adult-to-adult. A child seeking advice from a parent is natural. Talking to a professional such as a physician or psychiatrist or seeking advice on how to fix a plumbing leak is also natural. Asking around for recommendations regarding a reliable roofer is wise.

Following your *own* mind and inner promptings is important.

Gentleness and Serenity:

Gentleness and serenity is a unique state of being. While living among the various vulgarities of society, it's like carrying around a peaceful garden within your Beingness and sitting on a sun-warmed bench in the tranquil center of it.

Value and Priorities

Value is closely associated with having priorities lined up right. Understanding value has nothing to do with money or finances. The type of value that's related to wisdom has nothing to do with anything of a touchable nature, including money, real estate or mutual funds. We're talking about the *spiritual* value of good deeds, words and thoughts.

The twin quality of value is *priority*. Understanding value begets a natural sequential order of correct priorities in one's life. By making the Now the number-one priority, life is lived to the fullest and is loaded with rich experiences that would otherwise go unnoticed and, consequently, unappreciated. Living for tomorrow places one's consciousness on the future instead of the moment.

Living for tomorrow causes deep anxiety that, of itself, is a personality-altering emotion and keeps you from *living* today. In turn, this brings about stressed relationships and a warped perspective of the present. A preoccupation with tomorrow impedes an appreciation for the moment. Live for today. Be ready for tomorrow by living today. A preoccupation with tomorrow, next month or even the next moment keeps you from truly living.

Unconditional Goodness:

When you do things like giving your new gloves to someone who needs them without thinking or helping someone so automatically without realizing you're doing it you are practicing Unconditional Goodness. When it is automatic without seeing it as anything special, you are practicing Unconditional Goodness.

Respect:

Respect requires a true and deep respect for all of life. Many people claim to have this respect, yet few do because it means no prejudicial attitudes, no sexism, no racial, religious, or ethnic negativity. It means no hunting for sport, no environmental misdeeds, no littering and no environmental or social negative impact. The ramifications of respect stretch far and wide. From relationships to family, from the environment to cross-cultural reaches. Practicing this respect is done through both action and inaction - active and passive responses.

Passive respect is to allow others to litter without interfering or judging. Allow them their lives and accept their behavior as 'theirs', without judgment. Teach without teaching. Teach primarily by example and by sharing.

Active respect is picking up litter or planting a tree or helping another in some manner.

Of course, these are very simplistic examples just to exemplify the idea, yet respect for all life brings a multitude of benefits. Most noticeable of these is the absence of negative attitudes toward others and the presence of a childlike wonderment over all the beautifully intricate facets of nature. This wonderment is born of an appreciation of the vitality of life itself and the awareness of its exquisiteness. This wonderment presents continual opportunities for discovery by revealing diverse ways in which all living forces thrive through their interconnectedness to each other. This unique wonderment brings clarity to the fact that this glorious interconnectedness of life is no small matter, that it has no confining bounds. Rather, it begins within self and expands outward like a pond ripple widening its circle out into infinity.

A deep respect for life and the wonderment that accompanies it opens one's eyes to magnificent sights, it opens one's mind to nature's wisdom, where all species communicate through the common language of universal consciousness.

Attitude:

Most all of wisdom's qualities are some type of attitude or perspective.

These qualities instill incredible personal power, a gentle force that serenely rests within one's sacred Beingness.

These qualities of wisdom can, sadly, give an unacceptable impression of you to others. Allow for that possibility so that learning can take place.

Having unconditional acceptance can appear as being unemotional, insensitive and uncaring.

Patience and perseverance can be interpreted as your being a dreamer or holding onto an obsessive idea.

Silence can be perceived as ignorance or a type of apathy.

Wisdom is none of those!

There Is Only Light

We are all the Light. To know and be fully aware of the Light and what it *feels* like to be the Light is difficult when you are surrounded by nothing **but** Light. The question is, how to know yourself as the Light when you are amidst the Light.

There is darkness so we can experience the Light. We are afraid of the dark only if we choose to be. There is nothing to be afraid of, unless you decide that there is.

In order to experience anything at all, the exact opposite of it is needed.

You would be unable to know Warm without Cold, Up without Down, Fast without Slow, Left without Right, Here without There, Now without Then, Light without Dark.

What we perceive as Darkness is an aspect of the Light that has lowered its Light (vibrational frequency) to give us the opportunity to choose LOVE instead of Anything Else. LOVE and Thank the Darkness for this opportunity. Let your Light shine.

Be aware that there is no one to forgive; that there is no soul in all creation less perfect than you. Forgive if you *feel* the need to forgive. Realize LOVE is the purest form.

Know that the Beings we perceive as Dark have slowed down their vibration and become very heavy to do this thing that will seem so unloving and Dark. They will have to pretend to be something Dark even though they really are Light. Always remember who they really are; Beings of Light who have turned themselves Dark to give you an opportunity to LOVE.

If you react in fear and judgment instead of with LOVE, the Beings of Light who have turned themselves Dark may remain lost and you may even become lost until another soul shows you both the Light through LOVE. Always remember to LOVE and Thank "All That Is".

Chapter 8

Desires, Programs And Who Is In Charge
You Create Your Own Fate

Many people think that Man's fate is decided by someone up there. **But** this 'someone' simply makes available to every Man the most powerful energy in the Universe - an energy capable of shaping a Man's destiny and of creating whole new galaxies. This energy is called human thought.

One must become consciously aware of this phenomenon as well as just knowing that this is so - one must *feel* it.

How completely we are able to become aware of it, to *feel* and understand it, determines the degree to which the secrets of this vast Universe of ours unfold before us, the degree to which we perceive how its natural wonders work.

It is only the conscious awareness and acceptance of the energy of thought that will allow us to make our lives and the lives of our loved ones truly happy. And yet it is precisely a happy life that is predestined for Man on the Earth.

And so we are obliged to persuade ourselves of the indisputability of the following conclusions:

First: Man is a thinking being.

Second: The power of the energy of thought has no equal in the universe: everything we see, including ourselves, is created by the energy of thought.

We can name off millions of objects from a primitive hammer to a space ship, yet the appearance of each one of these is preceded by thought.

Our imagination builds a material object in space unseen to our eyes. It exists even though we have yet to glimpse its materialization. It is already constructed in mental space, and this is more significant than its subsequent materialization.

A space ship is constructed by the thought of one or more people. We still are unable to see it or touch it, yet at the same time it exists! It exists in a dimension invisible to us, **but** later it materializes, taking on a form we can see with our ordinary sight.

Which is more important in the construction of a space ship - the craftsmanship of the worker executing the details according to the blueprints presented to him, or the thought of the designer and builder? Of course the physical labor on any project is absolutely necessary, **but** nothing can displace the primacy of thought.

A real space ship can suffer a catastrophic accident which is always caused by an inadequately developed thought. In ordinary parlance it is known as thoughtlessness.

Thought is capable of foreseeing any kind of accident. In thought there are no unforeseen situations. Yet all sorts of accidents and irregularities do happen. Why? Because of haste in turning the project into material reality; rushing the thought process.

Anyone who thinks this through on their own can come to the same indisputable conclusion: all objects that have ever been manufactured on the Earth are materialized thoughts.

Now it is vitally necessary to realize that absolutely all life situations, including life itself, are formed first of all in thought.

The world of living Nature which we see, including Man himself, was originally formed by God's thought.

Just like God, Man is capable of forming with his thought his own life situations as well as new objects.

If your thought is insufficiently developed or prevented by some cause from freely making use of its inherent energy and speed capabilities, your life situations will be influenced by somebody else's thoughts - possibly the thoughts of your family, acquaintances, or society in general.

Note that even in this case your life situations are determined beforehand by human thought. And you have only yourselves to blame if you have choked and imprisoned your own thinking, thereby subjecting yourselves to the will of another person's thoughts. If you allow this, your successes or failures in life are dependent on other person or persons thoughts

You may be persuaded of what I have just said through a variety of examples in life. Think what a Man does before becoming a famous performing artist? First of all he dreams about it; then thinks up a plan of how to attain his dream and then steps into action. He takes part in amateur productions, studies at an appropriate school, and then takes a job in the theatre, film studio or symphony orchestra.

Some people may protest and say that while everybody dreams of becoming the most famous performing artist, only a few actually achieve this, while others are obliged to look for work in another field that has nothing to do with a career in the arts. Besides the dream, one needs talent too. Yes, of course, that is true. Realize that talent is also a product of the power of thought.

What about physical and natural gifts? They are significant, of course. Then again, human thought is wise enough to avoid inspiring a legless person to enroll in a ballet school.

How can it be, you may wonder: If everything, even one's profession and well-being, depended on one's own thoughts, then surely everybody would be rich and famous, and there would be no people eking out a pitiful existence, rummaging through garbage dumps in search of something to eat.

Adapted by author from Vladimir Megre, Book # 7: *The Energy Of Life,* pages 12 - 13 of The Ringing Cedars Series

Who Is In Charge?

In the excerpt below, Anastasia, a Siberian recluse is speaking to the author of *The Ringing Cedars of Russia* books. They met in the Taiga of northern Russia. She has a way of explaining things concisely and clearly and the section below totally resonates with me.

This conversation takes place between Anastasia and Vladimir after Vladimir's trip to Cyprus as described in Book #5: *Who Are We?* (p. 244 - 247) of The Ringing Cedars Series. In this section, I left Vladimir's use of the word ***not*** in places where it conveys his frustration and doubts.

"**But** there is no denying that there is a pattern to what has been happening, Vladimir," Anastasia calmly observed.

I *felt* my whole insides turn cold, and I was suddenly overwhelmed with some kind of extraordinary sense of apathy following these last words of Anastasia's. I did have a hope - a faint one, **but** still a hope - that she would be able to dissolve the whole *feeling* that had been building up in me of Man's utter insignificance - my insignificance and all mankind's. How could she have? Who would dare deny what is so patently obvious? Indifferent to everyone and everything, I stood by the window in a room lit only by moonlight, and looked out at the stars.

Somewhere out there, perhaps on one of those very stars, lived those who were controlling us, toying with us. *They* were living, *they* were real! **But** could *our* existence really be called life? A toy in subjugation to somebody's will can be said to live a dependent life - which meant only one thing: *we were **not** living.* This is why we are indifferent to so many things.

Once again Anastasia began talking in that same quiet and calm voice. **But** this time her voice left me unmoved and emotionless - it was more like some kind of extraneous sound.

"Vladimir, you and the people who sent you that cassette with the report were right: there really are energies out there capable of changing time, joining together into a single chain various events or, as happened with you, arranging a chain of circumstances required to achieve a predetermined goal. There is no such thing as pure coincidences - that is already clear to many people. Coincidences, even those which seem to be the most far-fetched, are programmed. Everything that happens to each individual is programmed. What happened to you on Cyprus, which served as a clear illustration for the researchers, as well as for you, was also programmed and then turned into reality.

"Tell me, please, Vladimir, would you like to know where the one directly responsible for programming your coincidences is now?"

"What difference does it make where he is? Does**n't** matter to me. On Mars, the Moon ... Whether he *feels* good or bad."

"He is right here in this room, Vladimir."

"That means, it's you?.. If so, that still doesn**'t** change anything. I'm **not** even surprised. And I'm **not** angry. I simply do**n't** care. We are manipulable, and that's the hopeless tragedy of the human race."

Vladimir. ..."I am able to exercise **but** a tiny speck of influence. The programmer is someone else."

"Then who *is* in charge? There's only two of us in the room. Or is there a third - a programmer who's invisible?"

"Vladimir, this programmer is right within you - it is *your desires.*"

"How so?"

"Only Man's desires and aspirations can launch any kind of program of action. This is the law of the Creator. Nobody, none of the energies of the Universe, can ever break that law. Because Man is the master of all the energies of the Universe! Man!"

"**But** I did **not** launch anything on Cyprus, Anastasia. Everything happened all by itself, by coincidence, apart from me."

"There were indeed certain minor incidents that were apart from the more significant events - though they contributed to their realization - and these incidents did happen apart from your will. **But** the basic events themselves were preceded by your desires. It was you who wanted to meet with the granddaughter of the goddess Aphrodite? You expressed your wish in the presence of witnesses and repeated it a number of times."

"Yes, I did ... "

"And if you remember that, then how can you call servants carrying out the will of their lord masters, and how can you call the master a plaything in their hands?"

"Yes, that *would* be silly. Interesting, how all this is turning out! Wow! Desires... **But** why then, are some of our desires left unfulfilled? Many people wish for things, **but** their wishes are unfulfilled. "

"So much depends on how meaningful the goal is. On whether the desire corresponds to the Light or the Dark. On how strong the desire is. The more substantial and bright the goal, the more the forces of light are drawn to fulfill it. To bring it about."

"And if the goal is a dark one - let's say, for example, to get drunk, or get into a fight, or plan a war? ... "

"Then the dark forces take over - Man through his desire has given them the opportunity to act. But, as you can see, it is still Man's desire that is first and foremost! Your desire, Vladimir."

I began to ponder what Anastasia had said, and my heart *felt* better and better. The very pleasant moonlight filled the whole room, and it seemed as though the stars in the sky were shining with a warm light where it had seemed cold. And Anastasia, sitting there on the edge of the bed, seemed to look even better than before. I said to her:

"You know, Anastasia, back there, when I first arrived on Cyprus, to be honest with you, I very nearly went on a binge. Because at first there seemed to be nothing I liked. Nobody spoke Russian. It was too noisy to work - people were whooping it up all around. *Why on earth did I end up here,* I thought, *maybe to get to know some hookers?* There are lots of women there, shall we say, of loose behavior - from both Russia and Bulgaria."

"You see, Vladimir? You had the desire, and there they were. You got drunk on vodka, and set up a date with them.

With one woman from Bulgaria, and another from Russia. Only even before that you wanted to meet with Aphrodite's granddaughter - your first desire proved to be stronger, and *she* appeared, and saved you from all the wretched stuff. She helped you."

"Yes, she did. And just how might you know about the Bulgarian girl?"

"From my *feelings*, Vladimir."

"I do**n't** understand that, **but** never mind. Tell me rather: this girl, Elena Fadeyeva, she's **not** the daughter of the goddess Aphrodite - she's Russian, she's simply an employee of a tourist agency on Cyprus. **But** I was talking about Aphrodite's granddaughter. Does that mean these forces of light were too puny to show me the real granddaughter of Aphrodite?"

"They are by no means 'puny'. And they did show you. The goddess Aphrodite today exists as energy. She is capable of connecting for a time with the energy of any Man - if she can see some meaningful reason to do so. Elena Fadeyeva, whenever she was with you, had two energies inside her. There was a lot she could do during those days. There was a lot she succeeded in doing, and she managed to help you, too."

"Yes, I'm grateful to her. *And* to the goddess Aphrodite." All my concerns and unpleasant sensations, connected with my assumption that all people were simply pawns in the hands of some kind of forces, literally flew out the window. Now, after my talk with Anastasia, a sense of confidence and peace set in.

Adapted by author from Vladimir Megre, Book # 5: *Who Are We?* (p. 244 - 247), The Ringing Cedars Series.

Naming Stars And Planets And Dogma

Below Anastasia , a Siberian recluse, is speaking to the author of "The Ringing Cedars of Russia" books. They met in the Taiga of northern Russia. She has a way of explaining things concisely and clearly and the section below totally resonates with me.

Anastasia talking to Vladimir

"Whenever you sleep under the stars, take your child with you, lay him down beside you, let him look at the stars. Under no circumstances tell him the names of the planets or how you perceive their origin and function, since this is something you only partially know yourself, and the dogmas stored in your brain will only lead the child astray from the truth. His subconscious knows the truth, and it will penetrate his consciousness all by itself. All you might do is to tell him that you like looking at the shining stars, and ask your child which star he likes best of all."

Planets, Astrology And Mans Thought

Below Anastasia , a Siberian recluse, is speaking to the author of "The Ringing Cedars of Russia" books. They met in the Taiga of northern Russia. She has a way of explaining things concisely and clearly and the section below totally resonates with me.

... I know that you find yourself unable to believe me at the moment - you are prevented from doing this by the conventions and many dogmas planted in your brain by the circumstances of existence in the world in which you live. The possibility of transport through time seems incredible to you. **But** your concepts of time and distance are all relative. These dimensions are beyond being measured by meters or seconds and can only be measured by the degree of one's conscious awareness and will.

The purity of the thoughts, *feelings* and perceptions held by the majority is what determines the place of humanity in time and the Universe.

You believe in horoscopes, you believe in your complete dependence on the position of the planets. This belief has been attained through the aid of the devices of the dark forces. This belief has been slowing down the movement of the channel of light, allowing its dark counterpart to advance and increase in size. This belief has been leading you away from a conscious awareness of the Truth, the essence of your earthly being. Analyze this question very carefully. Think about how God created Man in His image and likeness. Man has been granted the greatest of freedoms - the freedom to choose between the darkness and the light. Man has been given a soul. The whole visible world is subject to Man, and Man is free even when it comes to his relationship to God - to love Him or to turn his back on Him. Nobody and nothing can control Man apart from his own will. God wants Man's love in return for His love, **but** God wants the love of a free Man, perfect in His likeness.

God has created everything we can see, including the planets. They serve to guarantee the order and harmony of all life, including plants and animals. They also help human flesh, **but** there is no way they have power over Man's heart and mind. It is Man who controls *their* movements through his subconscious.

If a single individual wanted a second Sun to flare up in the sky, nothing would appear. Things are arranged this way to avoid planetary catastrophes. If everybody together wanted a second Sun, it would appear.

In making up a horoscope, it is necessary first of all to take into account the basic dimensions - the level of Man's temporal awareness, his strength of will and his spirit, the aspirations of his soul and the degree to which it participates in the life of the here and now.

Favorable and unfavorable astrological signs, magnetic storms, high and low pressure - these are all subject to will and conscious awareness.

Have you never seen a happy and joyful person on a cloudy or stormy day - or, on the other hand, a sad and depressed person on a sunny day with a most favorable astrological prediction?

Adapted by author from Vladimir Megre, Book # 1: *Anastasia,* pages 80 and 145 of The Ringing Cedars Series

Too Much Information

To find the right words, or to cite the examples needed for understanding, is a challenging task. Examples! Anastasia compared the modern computer to a prosthesis for the brain - in other words, to a prosthesis for thinking. It is probably true that people most familiar with how a computer works will understand and *feel* the importance of thinking speed more readily than others.

Below Anastasia , a Siberian recluse, is speaking to the author of "The Ringing Cedars of Russia" books. They met in the Taiga of northern Russia. She has a way of explaining things concisely and clearly and the section below totally resonates with me.

Anastasia speaking, "After all, you too, Vladimir, are able to work on a computer. Maybe through the computer you will be able to more quickly appreciate the catastrophic consequences of the sluggishness of human thinking.

Anyone familiar with a computer knows how important for the computer the size of its memory is and its operating speed. Note, I said: *operating speed.*

Now imagine what could happen if one were to slow down the operating speed of a computer controlling an aircraft's flight or a nuclear power plant. The computer might allow an accident to happen, and that would mean a disaster.

The living biological computer native to every Man on the Earth is incomparably more efficient than the manufactured variety. It is called upon to assist in the controlling of an immeasurably more perfect and massive device - the planets of the Universe.

These *can* be governed when this biological computer operates at a speed approximating or surpassing that of the original. However, the speed has been diminishing, and has continued to diminish. Anyone can see this for themselves if they **but** examine the situation more carefully.

When even the most state-of-the-art manufactured computer keeps getting loaded day by day, hour by hour, with all sorts of data - any kind of data as long as it is being inputted - eventually it will start to work more slowly, or it may refuse to process any new information whatsoever. This happens when its memory is overloaded to the point it can no longer accept new data.

Most people on the Earth today have experienced something like this. And the system created by the original priests (let go of religion) has got out of control. It has started operating all on its own.

When I mentioned earlier the monster devouring the children, I was talking about the system which has got out of control. Take a careful look:

When a child is born to an earthly mother, what is it that immediately takes it into its mighty clutches?

The system.

What determines what food is to be given to the child?

The system.

What determines what kind of air the child is to breathe and what kind of water he is to drink?

The system.

What determines the selection of his path in life?

The system.

Adapted by author from Vladimir Megre, Book # 7: *The Energy Of Life,* pages 58 and 59

Information Compressed In The Form Of Feelings

Below Anastasia , a Siberian recluse, is speaking to the author of "The Ringing Cedars of Russia" books. They met in the Taiga of northern Russia. She has a way of explaining things concisely and clearly and the section below totally resonates with me.

The following is a conversation between Anastasias' 9 year old son (Volodya) and Vladimir as in Book # 8.1: *The New Civilization* of The Ringing Cedars Series.

The son begins: "...And they (people) get confused in their life because they include no knowledge of life and no *feelings* capable of sensing God."

"**But** with Grandfather, all the information about the past, you're saying, has been retained?"

"Yes, Papa. Our Grandfather is a great priest and wise man. There is only one person living on the Earth today who significantly surpasses him in power."

"Where is he living right now, this strongest and wisest one - do you know? You must be talking about the high priest?"

"I am talking about our Mama Anastasia, Papa."

"Anastasia? **But** how could she have more information and greater knowledge than your great-grandfather?"

"Grandfather says he is hindered by too much information. And he can forget things. **But** Mama experiences no such hindrance, because there is no information contained in her."

"What do you mean? Which is it - does she really know more, or has she no knowledge at all?"

"I need to express myself more accurately, Papa. With Mama Anastasia all the information ... how shall I put it? .. she has a great deal more, only it is compressed in the form of *feelings*. And whenever she needs to, she is able to *feel* in a single moment something that Grandfather might require a day or two, or even more, to think about."

"I understand only part of what you've said, **but** it *is* interesting. Tell me more. What about you? Does this mean that you possess incomplete information about the past, seeing how you've had to consult with Grandfather?"

"That is correct."

"Why? You mean to say you're mentally inferior to them - Grandfather and Great-grandfather? And what do they tell you about this? Grandfather probably tells you that I'm to blame?"

"Grandfather never told me anything like that."

"**But** what about Mama? What did she say?"

"I asked Mama why I know less than my forebears. And less than she, or even you, Papa. And this was her answer:

"'All the truths of the Universe, son, and all the information accumulated right from its pristine origins, has always been available to every Man, nothing hidden. Some people are incapable of understanding it and making it their own, because their life-goals and the aspirations of their souls are out of harmony with those of the Universe. Man has free will in everything, and is free to choose a path other than that of the Universe. God is free too, as to when, how and to whom He gives a hint. You must let go of worry about information that is lacking in you. Seek out your dream and know that the whole will be offered to you in full, if the dream that is born within you is worthy of co-creation.'"

"Hmmm... So tell me, Volodya, what do *you* make of all that?"

"Once my dream and life-goal are created in all their detail, all the knowledge I need to turn the dream into reality will be born in me all on its own, without fail."

"**But** in the meantime, then, you will go on consulting with Grandfather?"

"Yes, with Grandfather, and Mama, and you, and I shall try to ponder life all on my own."

Adapted by author from Vladimir Megre, Book # 8.1: *The New Civilization,* pages 46 and 47 of The Ringing Cedars Series

Personal Notes

_____

_____

_____

_____

_____

_____

_____

_____

_____

_____

_____

_____

Chapter 9
Healing Vs. Curing And Knowing When To Step Back
Healing Vs. Curing

Is it best to eliminate *all* diseases and remove *all* challenges for others or even yourself?"

Healing of physical ailments can bring harm to someone. Modern doctors and many healers typically think that curing someone is always a good thing and ignore the underlying causes of the ailment, which lie in their patients' souls and the souls plan for this lifetime.

Working against the person's spiritual interests is something that needs to kept in mind.

Below Anastasia , a Siberian recluse, is speaking to the author of "The Ringing Cedars of Russia" books. They met in the Taiga of northern Russia. She has a way of explaining things concisely and clearly and the section below totally resonates with me. She healed a woman and was told by her grandfather that she had made a mistake.

"My grandfather showed me an example of the harm that healing can bring when it is inadequately thought through, when the patient is a bystander instead of a participant in the healing."

I decided to help a woman, and one night when she lay down to sleep I began warming her with my Ray, removing the pains from her body. I could *feel* some kind of resistance to the Ray, **but** I still kept on trying. I did this for about ten minutes until I succeeded in healing her flesh.

Then, when Grandfather came, I told him about the old woman, and I asked him why the Ray had met some resistance. He thought about it, and then told me I had done the wrong thing. It made me very distraught.

I began asking Grandfather to explain why. At first he was silent. Then he said, 'You healed the body.'"

Anastasia then continues:

"The woman's health got better and she lived. Her son came to see her earlier than usual. This time he came only for two days and told his mother he had quit his studies and had no desire to be an artist any more. He was now involved in some other work that brought in more money. He had got married. Now he would have a lot of money, and he no longer wanted her to prepare 'those insipid food jars' for him, since transporting them would now cost more.

'You can eat better yourself, now, Mother', he said.

He left without taking anything. That morning the woman sat on her porch, looked at her plot, and her eyes were filled with such emptiness and depression — they looked as though she had lost the will to live. You see, her body was healthy, **but** it was as if there were no life left in it. I saw, or rather *felt*, the terrible emptiness and hopelessness in her heart.

If I had allowed the natural flow instead of curing her body, the woman would have died at the right time, she would have died peacefully with her beautiful dream and hope intact. Now here she was, still alive, **but** in great despair, and this was many times more frightening than physical death.

Two weeks later she passed on." Adapted by author from Vladimir Megre, Book # 2: *The Ringing Cedars of Russia,* pages 23-26 of The Ringing Cedars Series

Helping When It Is Against Natural Universal Laws

Below Anastasia, a Siberian recluse is speaking to the author of "The Ringing Cedars of Russia" books. They met in the Taiga of northern Russia. She has a way of explaining things concisely and clearly and the section below totally resonates with me.

The following conversation between Anastasia and Vladimir took place while Vladimir was being guided by Anastasia and remotely viewing. A family being robbed and assaulted in their home came into Vladimir's awareness.

Vladimir cried out to Anastasia, "Go back! Do something!"

She went back to the scene and replied:

"I have to respect the laws of choice. It has already happened. It is too far along. It should have been stopped earlier, **but** now it is too late."

"Do something!" Vladimir cried to Anastasia. "If you have any heart at all, do at least something!"

"It is beyond my power. Everything has been, so to speak, programmed in advance. The choices have already been made by those involved. No one, including me, should interfere directly. They have the upper hand right now."

"**But** where's that goodness of yours - your powers?"

"I tried to fulfill your request," she quietly said, and a minute later added: "I think I succeeded."

"**But** you look so bad - you almost died!"

I violated the natural laws. I interfered in something I should have left alone. That required all my strength and energy. I am surprised that they held out at all."

"Why did you take such a risk, if you knew it was so dangerous?"

"I had no choice - After all, you wanted me to do something. **I was afraid** that if I refused to fulfill your request, you would lose all respect for. me. You would think that all I can do is talk, that I am all words ... And that I could do nothing in real life."

Her eyes looked at me enquiringly and pleadingly. Her soft voice trembled a little as she spoke.

"The explanation of how to do it, how this natural system works is beyond spoken words. _I feel it._ It is beyond my ability to explain to you, in a way you could understand, and it is probable your scholars will be unable to explain it."

"So what can be done? What can you suggest, apart from pitying them?"

"They can only be helped through increasing their sincere, spiritual communication with each other. They need to strive, with complete sincerity, for purity of thought."

Adapted by author from Vladimir Megre, Book # 1: *Anastasia,* pages158 -161 of The Ringing Cedars Series

Unknowingly Preventing Someone From Experiencing Something That Was Necessary For Their Souls Growth.

When you help people and do the work for them you can unknowingly prevent them from an experience that was necessary for their souls growth.

When you see someone or several people who are about to get their heads bashed in or shot, is it always best to help them?

Is it best that the spirit still fighting in them takes care of the situation?

What can they do against thugs with guns?

Is it best that you intervene or would it be interfering with their souls growth and highest good?

As long as their spirit is still fighting, nobody should interfere. Assistance **may be** appropriate. Outside interference may take care of the situation at hand, **but** it will weaken their self-confidence, and mean that a whole lot of other situations in their lives will turn out unfavorably for them. They will come to rely on outside help.

Instead of telling someone what you see as an outcome, encourage and allow them to see and *feel* their own outcome through their connection to Divinity/Great Spirit.

Leave Your Friends Alone

Too often instead of working on our own changes, we decide which of our friends or acquaintances needs to change. This is *our resistance* and is a type of interference.

In the early days of my work, I had a client who would send me to all her friends in the hospital. Instead of sending them flowers, she would have me go to fix up their problems. I would arrive with my tape recorder in hand, usually finding someone in bed who had no idea why I was there or understood what I was doing. This was before I learned never to work with anyone unless he or she requested it.

Sometimes clients come to me because a friend has given them a session as a present. This usually has a poor outcome, and they seldom come back for further work.

When something works well for us, we often want to share it with others. **But** they may need time before they are ready to make a change. It's hard enough to make changes when we want to, **but** to try to make someone else change when he or she is unwilling is impossible, and it can ruin a good friendship. I push my clients because they come to me. I leave my friends alone.

Adapted by author from Louise Hay, *You Can Heal Your Life,* page 56

Healing The Past, Present And Future Explained

You heal your past and future incarnations, your ancestry and your descendants as you heal your-self in the present moment. As you heal your ancestry you also help to heal the rest of your family, including brothers, sisters, cousins, nieces and nephews. There is no time, place or space except as we create and perceive it. If what you are healing is in a parallel universe as you perceive it, healing is done in the same manner. Time and space are immaterial except that they help us process as humans.

Realize, know and be aware that as you heal your-self there is a ripple effect that helps 'All That Is' to heal. **This includes all aspects of your-self in all we perceive as dimensions, realities and times.** This in some measure goes to infinity.

A person's meridians and energy centers and earths grid system are interconnected and affect each other

Healing the Past, Present And Future Charts

Healing the Past

\# = Number of lifetimes or generations into the Past.

Me = Me in this lifetime.   M = mother.   F = father

You may sometimes need to know who you are healing for. It may be further back than this chart goes.

As you become aware of who and what you are healing, ask, "Is it best if I know more?".

Once there there is no need to know more any more investigation is for curiosity and may bring in ego.

Remamber, you are healing yourself.   Allow others their own path..

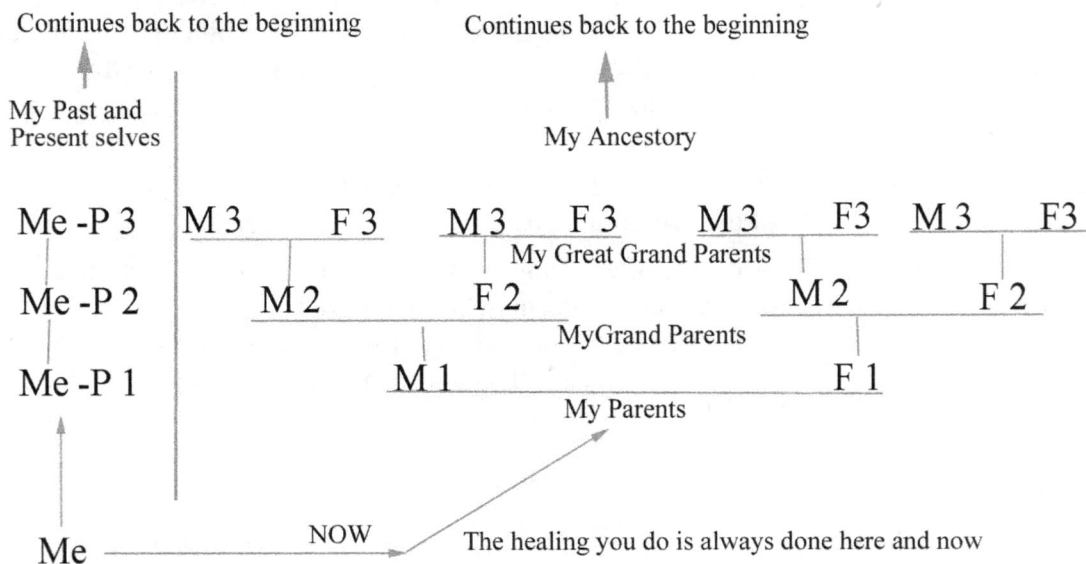

Continues back to the beginning   Continues back to the beginning

My Past and Present selves   My Ancestory

| Me -P 3 | M 3 | F 3 | M 3 | F 3 | M 3 | F 3 | M 3 | F 3 |

My Great Grand Parents

| Me -P 2 | M 2 | F 2 | M 2 | F 2 |

MyGrand Parents

| Me -P 1 | M 1 | F 1 |

My Parents

Me ———— NOW ———— The healing you do is always done here and now

Healing the Future

\# = Number of lifetimes or generations into the Future.

Me = Me in this lifetime.
D = daughter

W or H = Wife or Husband
S = son

You may sometimes need to know who you are healing for. It may be further forward than this chart goes.

As you become aware of who and what you are healing, ask, "Is it best if I know more"?

Once there there is no need to know more any more investigation is for curiosity and may bring in ego.

As you Heal Yourself, You Help Your Desendants To Heal If They Choose To.

If Your Wife or Husband Heals Themselves That Also Helps Your Desendants To Heal

Remember, you are healing yourself.   Allow others their own path.

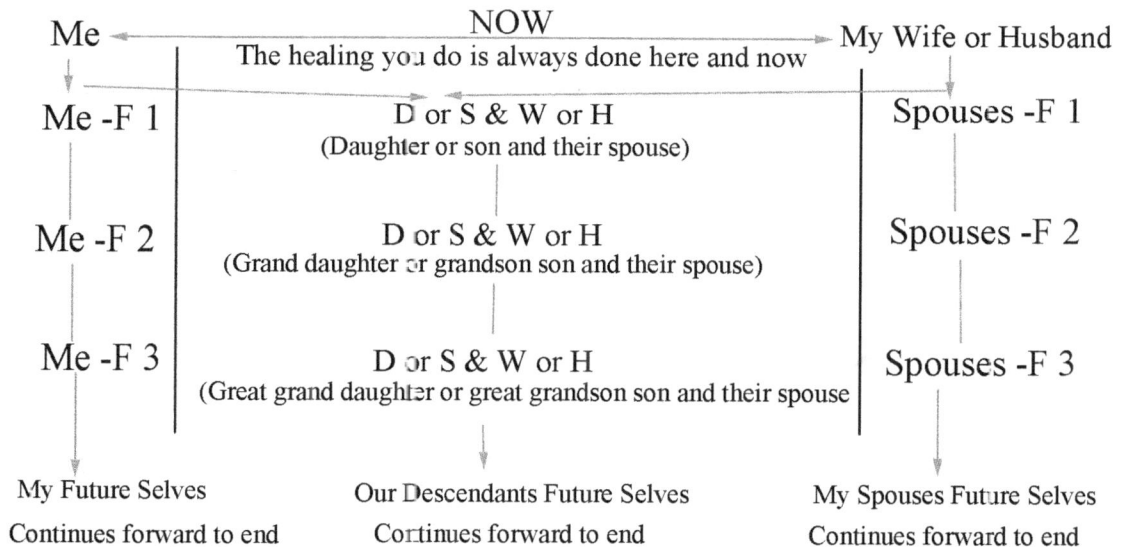

	NOW	
Me ←	The healing you do is always done here and now →	My Wife or Husband
Me -F 1	D or S & W or H (Daughter or son and their spouse)	Spouses -F 1
Me -F 2	D or S & W or H (Grand daughter or grandson son and their spouse)	Spouses -F 2
Me -F 3	D or S & W or H (Great grand daughter or great grandson son and their spouse	Spouses -F 3
My Future Selves	Our Descendants Future Selves	My Spouses Future Selves
Continues forward to end	Continues forward to end	Continues forward to end

Personal Notes

Chapter 10

Receiving Your Own Information And Guidance Through *Feeling*

Practice Feeling

Calm and center yourself the best you can. Make the clearest connection to Great Spirit you can.

Then say to yourself silently,

"In this life time and in this physical body, my name is __make something up__". (if you are looking at a wall or tree you could say "wall" or "tree"). Before you even finish mentalizing what you are going to say, start paying attention to how you *feel* and what you sense. You may sense, *feel* or even see a restriction somewhere in your body or energy field and *feel* more tense.

Let go of the above *feeling* and now say to yourself silently,

"In this life time and in this physical body, my name is __say your name__". Before you even finish mentalizing what you are going to say, start paying attention to how you *feel* and what you sense. You may sense, *feel* or even see a relaxation somewhere in your body or energy field and *feel* more relaxed and happy.

With practice you will be more and more able to *feel* the same sensations when you have a thought, when you are reading, when you are watching TV and even when you are having a normal conversation or working. Learn to recognize this as a form of intuition and guidance.

As you practice, there are ways to confirm whether something is true or false; of LOVE or Anything Else. Some of the ways are through kinesiology (muscle testing), use of a pendulum, a mental chalk board and several other forms of autonomic response testing.

Good information on Muscle testing at <http://www.holistichealthtools.com/muscle.html>.

Your Body As A Source Of Awareness

You can use your body as a source of awareness without taking things into your body.

Learn to listen to your body. Allow your body to tell you what is good for it and good for you. When you go against your knowing *feeling*, or your body, you will create illness or something else in your body. Your body will let you know if you are going to the wrong place!

Light Vs. Heavy:

Does it *feel* heavy or light?

It's a universal law that what is true *feels* light, while anything that *feels* heavy is untrue for you. How does it *feel* to you? If it *feels* heavy at all, it is of something other than LOVE and TRUTH.

Thought

Is the thought that's making me heavy actually mine?

If you get a sense of lightening up anyplace in your universe when you ask this question, it is someone else's thought in the first place.

If it is yours, investigate with awareness instead of thought and **heal, transmute, release and integrate it.**

If it's someone else's, say from the heart:

All layers return to sender with full consciousness and Divine Love.

Pain

Be aware that pain is emotional and mental as well as physical. You can even ask, "Is this my thought or fear?"

"Body, what are you trying to tell me with this pain?"

"Is this my pain? (Even if it is intense)

If you're sure the pain is actually yours—if it stays heavy, without lightning for even a nanosecond it yours. If the pain lightens up even for a nanosecond when you ask the question, "Is this my pain?", **it is** someone else's. Even if it comes back after initially lightening up when you asked the question, it still may be someone else's; it merely means you have bought the lie that it is yours. The way to handle this is to transmute and un-create all your decisions to buy the pain as yours when it was someone else's.

If it is yours, investigate with awareness instead of thought, and heal, transmute and release it, and then integrate the positive.

If it's someone else's ask:

"Is it best I know who this pain belongs to?"

> **If yes:** ask: who's pain it is before sending it back with LOVE and compassion, asking Great Spirit to assist them in dealing with and healing it as is best.
> **If no:** send it back with LOVE and compassion, asking Great Spirit to assist whoever's it is in dealing with and healing it as is best.

Chapter 11

Life Long Effects Of Prenatal And Perinatal Experiences (Including Toxins) And Vanishing Twins

Introduction To Information On Prenates And Vanishing Twins

This section is included because I *feel* strongly that the unborn child, from the time of conception to shortly after birth is especially susceptible to the *feelings* and emotions of the mother and to a slightly lesser extent the father, siblings and family. I also *feel* the most powerful time for the unborn child to take on emotions of the mother and father is when the blastocyst implants into the uterine wall on about day 6 after floating in the uterus for a day or two. Direct physical contact with the mother is the first time there is no filter between the mother's *feelings* and the unborn child's.

Identical (monozygotic) twins are formed when one egg and one sperm become a single zygote. With identical twins, it is the zygote that divides into two embryos. This usually occurs between 3-8 days after fertilization and the embryos will have one placenta and two amniotic sacs. Sometimes it will occur before this time and each will have their own placenta and sac. Less frequently, the zygote will split up until 13 days post-conception with the embryos sharing a single sac and placenta. Complications are more likely in this case. Rarely, the split will occur after this, resulting in conjoined, or Siamese, twins.

Fraternal (dizygotic) twins are always two zygotes. A sperm and egg become a zygote and a second sperm and second egg become a second zygote.

More detailed information follows.

Prenatal (in the womb):

Conception:

> First the sperm and egg combine to form a Zygote.

Zygote (approximately days 0 to 5):

> The earliest developmental stage of the embryo in multi cell organisms. When a single sperm enters the mother's egg cell, the resulting cell is called a zygote. The zygote contains all of the genetic information (DNA) needed to become a baby. Half of the genetic information comes from the mother's egg and half from the father's sperm. The zygote spends the next few days (about 3 days) traveling down the Fallopian tube and divides to form a ball of cells before entering the uterus.

Blastocyst (approximately days 5 to 10):

> The zygote continues to divide, creating an inner group of cells with an outer shell. This stage is called a blastocyst. The inner group of cells will become the embryo, while the outer group of cells will become the membranes that nourish and protect it.
> The blastocyst reaches the womb (uterus) around day 5, and implants into the uterine wall on about day 6. At this point in the mother's menstrual cycle, the lining of the uterus has grown and is ready to support a baby.

Implantation on the uterine wall at about day 6 up to day 10:

> The blastocyst sticks tightly to the lining, where it receives nourishment via the mother's bloodstream.

Embryo (approximately weeks 2 to 7):

> The cells of what is now an embryo multiply and begin to take on specific functions. This process is called differentiation. It leads to the various cell types that make up a human being (such as blood cells, kidney cells, and nerve cells).
>
> There is rapid growth, and the baby's main external features begin to take form. It is during this critical period (most of the first trimester) that the growing baby is most susceptible to damage. The following can interfere with the baby's development:
>> 1)Alcohol, certain prescription and recreational drugs, and other substances that cause birth defects
>>
>> 2)Infection (such as rubella or cytomegalovirus)
>>
>> 3)Nutritional deficiencies
>>
>> 4)X-rays or radiation therapy

The end of the 10th week of pregnancy marks the end of the "embryonic period" and the beginning of the "fetal period."

> Fetus (approximately week 8 to birth):

Adapted by author from *<http://umm.edu/health/medical/ency/articles/fetal-development>*.

Perinatal (Shortly before birth; the birth process itself and shortly after birth)

> The Perinatal period is defined in diverse ways. Depending on the definition, it starts at the 20th to 28th week of gestation and ends 1 to 4 weeks after birth.

Vanishing Twins

> A loss of one twin during pregnancy can occur in the first trimester (often before the mother even knows she's carrying twins) or less commonly, later in the pregnancy.
>
> Documented rates of vanishing twin syndrome have grown significantly over the past few decades, as early ultrasounds have become routine. Overall, the rate of the loss of one twin is probably around 20 to 30 percent. Often there are no symptoms at all.

The Vulnerable Prenate

Introduction

The prenate (i.e., the unborn baby) is vulnerable in a number of ways that are generally unrecognized and unarticulated. Most people think or assume that prenates are unaware, and seldom attribute to them the status of being human. I recall a recent train trip, where an expectant mother sat in a smoking car filled with boisterous and noisy people. I asked her whether she had any concern for her unborn baby, and whether she thought the smoke or the noise would be bothersome to her unborn child. Her reply was, "No way, my dear. Their intelligence is very limited and they are asleep so to speak." Nothing could be further from the truth. Theory and research from the last 20 years indicates that prenatal experiences can be remembered, and have lifelong impact. The major purpose of this article is to clarify the conditions under which prenatal experiences may lead to lifelong problems and challenges, and to describe the theoretical and research perspectives that are necessary to understand the effects of prenatal traumatization.

Interactional Trauma

The effects of prenatal traumatization can only be predicted with knowledge of other factors, and prenatal experiences are likely to have lifelong impact when they are followed by reinforcing conditions or interactional trauma. The term interactional trauma means that traumas interact with each other in producing their effects. In statistical analyses, interactional means that the effects of factors depend on the presence of other factors. Both of these definitions communicate the meaning of interaction as it is used in this article. For example, it is unlikely that being stuck during the birthing process causes claustrophobia during adulthood. However, claustrophobia is more likely if similar reinforcing traumas occur later in life..

In one such case that I treated, a baby who had been stuck during his birth was also locked in a closet for 24 hours as a child, and held and choked by his brother on several occasions. Several points are relevant here. First of all, prenatal traumas provide 'tinctures" for later experiences. Stated differently, life experiences are perceived in terms of prior and unresolved traumas. When a baby is stuck during birth, the baby is likely to perceive later events as entrapping, or to unconsciously manipulate or choose life situations that bring about entrapment. This process is called recapitulation. Secondly, similar or recapitulated events, independent of perceptual processes, are likely to reinforce prenatal traumas, resulting in relatively chronic symptoms. In the case of the baby just described, childhood events acted as reinforcements for the birth trauma, resulting in chronic claustrophobia.

The Effects Of Prenatal Experiences: Prenates Are Conscious Aware Beings

During the 1995 APPPAH Congress in San Francisco, David Chamberlain shared a case that exemplifies the consciousness of prenates. In this case, a baby was undergoing amniocentesis (A test that detects chromosomal abnormalities in the fetus. A sample of amniotic fluid is taken from the amniotic sac (amnion) surrounding the unborn baby and its DNA is examined). Videotapes of the amniocentesis showed that when the needle was inserted into the uterus, the baby turned toward the needle and batted it away. Thinking that they had seen an aberration, medical staff repeated the needle insertion, and again, the baby batted the needle away. There are other anecdotal reports that babies routinely withdraw from needles as they are inserted into the uterus. From these observations, it is safe to conclude that babies are very conscious of what is happening around them, particularly with respect to events that have impact on them personally.

In her book *From Fetus to Child*, Alessandra Piontelli cites several cases of prenatal awareness. She describes a twin pair, at about four months of gestation, who were very conscious of each other, and had periodic interactions. One of the twins was actively aggressive, the other submissive. Whenever the dominant twin was pushing or hitting, the submissive twin withdrew and placed his head on the placenta, appearing to rest there. In life, when these twins were four years of age, they had the same relationship. Whenever there was fighting or tension between the pair, the passive twin would go to his room and put his head on his pillow. He also carried a pillow and used it as his "security blanket,' resting on it whenever his twin became aggressive. From this and other research (such as David Chamberlain's Babies Remember Birth, and

Elizabeth Noble's Primal Connections), it seems clear that prenates are conscious beings and that behaviors that begin in utero are also likely to carry over into later life.

Prenatal Events Are Remembered

For years, it was hard to understand how prenatal experiences could be remembered. The central nervous system is very rudimentary during the prenatal period, and there is a myelination process which continues through childhood. Until then, nerves and the nervous system are only partially protected be a developing myelin sheath. However, anecdotal reports of adults regressed to the prenatal period and remembering prenatal events are common in primal and regressive communities. In 1970 Graham Farrant, an Australian medical doctor, began experiencing prenatal events and recording his body experiences. He was quite astonished to discover that he experienced most of his significant prenatal memories at a cellular rather than a tissue or skeletal-muscular level, and he referred to his recollections as cellular memory. In 1975 Frank Lake, an English theologian and psychiatrist, found that prenatal memories stemmed from viral cells, that viruses were primitive prenatal cells that formed during trauma and carried traumatic memories. He consistently referred to prenatal memories in terms of cellular memories. Over the last five years, there has been a considerable amount of research done in cellular biology, all of it supporting the theory that memories can be encoded in cells. The research of Dr. Bruce Lipton, reported in the 1995 APPPAH Congress, is relevant here and supports the conclusions of Farrant and Lake.

Prenatal Memories May Be The Most Influential

A group of European psychologists, led by R. D. Laing and Frank Lake (both now deceased), contend that prenatal memories are the most influential because they are the first. This perspective is apparent in Laing's book, *The Facts of Life*, where he writes, "The environment is registered from the very beginning of my life; by the first one (cell) of me. What happens to the first one or two of me may reverberate throughout all subsequent generations of our first cellular parents. That first one of us carries all my 'genetic' memories". He goes on to say, "It seems to me credible, at least, that all our experience in our life cycle, from cell one, is absorbed and stored from the beginning, perhaps especially in the beginning. How can that happen. How can one cell generate the billions of cells I now am? We are impossible, **but** for the fact that we are. When I look at the embryological stages in my life cycle, I experience what *feel* to me like sympathetic vibrations in me now...how I now *feel* I *felt* then". Frank Lake mirrored Laing's perspectives. Lake contended that the most formative experiences were ones that occurred prenatally, especially during the first trimester. In the U.S., Lloyd deMause has also written about the social, cultural and political influences of prenatal experiences, and reported on these findings during the 1995 APPPAH Congress.

Prenates Incorporate Parental Experiences And *Feelings*

From his regressions with adult patients, Lake also found that the most influential events were maternal experiences that passed biochemically through the umbilical cord by means of a group of chemicals called catecholamines. It is also true that prenates incorporate psychic prenatal *feelings* and experiences, especially those of their mothers. Maternal emotions (and paternal emotions through the mother's emotional response to them) infiltrate the fetus. Research shows that what mothers experience, babies also experience. A good example is the following case. A woman's father died just prior to the conception of her child. She spent the whole nine months *feeling* depressed and grieving the loss of her father. If it is true that babies experience and remember what their mothers experience, then her baby should also have experienced loss and depression, and these *feelings* would be expected to resurface during childhood and/or adulthood. This appeared to be the case.

As a child, her baby was periodically depressed, and medical personnel could find no physiological or psychological basis for the depression (They were unaware of the child's prenatal experiences). When the child was depressed, he would draw pictures of old and dying men in caves (in prenatal and perinatal psychology, caves are symbolic of wombs, the place where he experienced the loss of his grandfather). After drawing, he would *feel* better for a while, **but** the depression would slowly return. He was unaware of any connection between his drawings and his grandfather's death. The depression became chronic when his parents were experiencing tension (his mother and father were living separately **but** raising him together). The tension symbolized the loss of his father and grandfather. His drawings sometimes depicted a little girl frantically searching for dying men. The little girl probably represented his own feminine, the mother's inner child, and/or a female twin's experience of the grandfather's loss. It is unlikely that grief would have resurfaced as chronic depression without the reinforcing conditions of father loss and parental discord. It is important to realize that although prenates do take on the prenatal experiences of their parents, they also have their own unique experiences during the prenatal period, independent of their parents. The mechanisms of how this works are becoming more clear through numerous anecdotal reports, and clinical cases show that prenates have their own experiences. For example, I recall the reports of a regressed child, a twin, who was repeatedly subjected to verbal and physical fights between his mother and her boyfriend during the prenatal period. He reported that his mother and her boyfriend were constantly fighting, **but** he and his twin would respond to this by cuddling up and rocking while the fighting went on. During the fighting, they both felt quite clever (to have avoided the tension) and relaxed. Perhaps the presence of a comforting twin can make it easier to separate from parental experiences easier.

When Reinforced, Prenatal Experiences May Have Dramatic And Symptomatic Influences

In the case of the woman who lost her father just prior to pregnancy, the baby presumably experienced the same loss that his mother experienced. In addition, a very tangible and personal trauma happened shortly thereafter. Early in the pregnancy, when she was eight weeks pregnant, the mother's husband abruptly left her for another woman. She was shocked by the experience and *felt* deeply abandoned. Presumably her unborn child *felt* abandoned as well. Because the woman had little financial security and *felt* she was unable to raise a child by herself, she decided to abort her child.

She attempted several abortions, most often by using the hooked or curved end of a coat hanger. As a child, her baby was periodically sadistic and self-destructive. The manifestations of his sadism bore a striking resemblance to his mother's abortion attempts, although he was consciously unaware of them. He burned himself with cigarettes and gouged private parts of his body with sharp metal objects. His favorite sadistic instrument was a fishing hook, **but** he complained he could never buy ones that were big enough. As a young adult he was arrested thirty times for assault, and his modus operandi was reminiscent of his mother's attempts to abort him. He usually assaulted his victims when they were sleeping, by using heavy braided wire with a wire hook welded on the end!

Aggression And Violence Are Pathological Symptoms Resulting From Multiple, Reinforcing Traumas With Themes Of Loss, Abandonment, And Aggression

In the case just described, the prenate experienced the intense loss and abandonment that his mother experienced. In addition, he also experienced the abandonment that comes with parental narcissism, (i.e., his mother was so absorbed in her abandonment and loss that she had little or no cognizance of him, nor did she have time or energy to celebrate his presence). On the contrary, he was perceived as a burden, and as something to get rid of. Consequently, he also experienced the aggression of his mother's abortion attempts on his life.

Prenatal And Birth Traumas Are Mirror Images

Prenatal traumas have two distinct impacts on birth. First of all, birth is often perceived and experienced in terms of prenatal traumatization. For example, babies who experience abortion attempts are also likely to experience birth as annihilative. Babies who experience near-death during implantation in the womb are likely to experience birth as a near-death experience. Babies who experience aggression or violence while in the womb are likely to experience the interventions of birth as aggressive and violent, even though there may be no such intent on the part of medical personnel or parents.

Secondly, as Sheila Kitzinger has documented, whenever there is significant prenatal stress (trauma), there is an increasing statistical likelihood that birth complications will occur. The greater the degree of stress or trauma during the prenatal period, the greater the likelihood of birth complications and obstetrical interventions. This is exactly what occurred in case of the mother whose father died just before she became pregnant, and who attempted several abortions. The mother had a very difficult birth with long labor and many complications. Many interventions were used and repeated, among which were inductions, augmentations, sedations, analgesias, anesthesias, forceps, episiotomy, intensive care placement, and respiration.

It should be pointed out that the severity of symptoms in the above case is due to the additional and reinforcing traumas, all involving loss, abandonment, and aggression. When the baby was three months old, the mother took him shopping in a stroller, forgot that he was with her, left him in an aisle of the store, and only realized her error hours later. In addition to this, she had a boyfriend who was repeatedly and physically abusive with her son during his early childhood. These multiple and reinforcing traumas manifested in his childhood and adulthood as aggression and violence.

Prenatal And Birth Traumas Impair Bonding At Birth

In addition to posing a risk of birth traumatization, prenatal traumas have another and more insidious impact. When traumas occur prior to or during birth, the quantity and quality of bonding is radically reduced. This reduction occurs for two reasons. The first has to do with the defensive dulling of mind and body, which is a natural defense. This self-anesthetization occurs because of the hormonal changes that normally occur in the body during and after trauma and shock. When the body and mind are dulled, and when the body is exhausted from stress, the quantity and quality of bonding are lessened.

The second impact has to do with the failure of parents and others to acknowledge traumatization, which diminishes the bonding process even further. When traumas occur, there is a critical period of time afterward during which humans require understanding, acknowledgment, and compassion in order for shock to subside and healing to begin. However, it is rare for babies to receive understanding, acknowledgment, and compassion after their prenatal and birth traumas, simply because no one knows or believes that traumas have taken place. As has been verified in my own clinical research with babies, unacknowledged traumas create distrust in babies, and this significantly impedes the bonding process. In contrast, it is informative to witness the level and depth of bonding in babies who have had no traumatic *feelings*, or whose traumatization is being seen and acknowledged. The bonding is noteworthy by its depth, intensity, and duration. One only has to witness such bonding to realize that bonding is significantly reduced and altered by the presence of unacknowledged and unresolved traumatization.

Lack Of Bonding Predisposes The Individual To Aggression And Violence

In my work with infants over the past 25 years, I have discovered some important interrelationships between prenatal trauma, birth trauma, bonding, and aggression. The first interrelationship is that birth, as has recently been practiced, actively impairs the bonding process because many aspects of the birthing process are psychologically and physically painful for babies. Medical exams and medical tests are often experienced by babies as unnecessary, invasive, and painful, and this is rarely acknowledged. Medical personnel routinely separate babies from parents after birth, and separation is often experienced as terrifying abandonment. Placement in intensive care is frequently experienced as terrifying, lonely, over-stimulating, and painful abandonment. Anesthetization is particularly impactful on bonding because residual amounts of anesthesia are common in babies, even hours and days after birth, and anesthesia makes babies (and mothers) numb and therefore less available to the bonding process. Epidurals were thought to be superior to other anesthetics because they would inhibit the bonding process less, **but** research shows that mothers who receive epidurals show less attachment to their babies than mothers who do without. These are some examples of the effects of birth trauma on bonding. In all cases bonding is affected because it is difficult for babies to trust their parents when their parents inaccurately perceive or leave the prenatal and birth traumas unacknowledged. In general, the greater the number and severity of unacknowledged prenatal and birth traumas, the greater the impact on bonding.

Secondly, when traumas are largely untreated, the influence on bonding is exacerbated because the traumatized infant remains in a defensive stance with respect to the world, and "keeps the world from touching him." Many parents report to me that their babies are very independent, **but** this is often a cover for defensiveness. Such babies act as if they are OK and have no need for comforting or support. They resist letting themselves be comforted and held, either pushing their parents away and/or ignoring their attempts to comfort and console them. Many times they will only let their parents comfort them after considerable resistance. Third, it is important to realize that a lack of bonding may be sufficient, in and of itself, to create aggression and violence. This surprising fact has been brought to light by various researchers. For example, Magid and McKelvey (1988) reported that children with severe bonding difficulties fail to develop a conscience, and perform asocial or antisocial acts without remorse. Felicity De Zulueta (1993) summarized research in the field of bonding and attachment, and concluded that violent aggression can be the result of damaged bonding. She writes, "One of the most important outcomes of...studies on attachment behavior is the emerging link between psychological trauma, such as loss (of a bond)...and destructive or violent behavior." She concludes that the more damage that is done to bonding, the greater the likelihood of aggression and violence during childhood and adulthood. Fourth, it is clear from the observations of clinical researchers that the probability of societal aggression and violence are increased greatly by the presence of aggression or violence during the prenatal and perinatal periods of development. Prenates pick up on aggressive and violent energies, and are likely to repeat what they experience in their prenatal life space.

What Kinds Of Prenatal And Perinatal Experiences Underline Aggression and Violence?

As a way of determining the prenatal, etiological bases for violence and aggression, I posed a basic question to a number of experts in the field, among whom were R. D. Laing, Frank Lake, Barbara Valassis, Barbara Findelsen, Stan Grof, Michael Irving, and others. I asked them to report on the kinds of regressive experiences that their aggressive and violent patients had uncovered and/or reported, and that were central in the success of treatment. Among their varied responses were common threads of consensus, among which were: (1) prenatal and perinatal experiences were paramount in aggression and violence; (2) childhood experiences seemed to reflect and reinforce prenatal traumatization; (3) aggression and violence were related to the severest levels of prenatal and perinatal trauma; (4) consistently related to aggression and violence were themes of loss, abandonment, rejection, and aggression; and (5) certain prenatal and perinatal traumas were consistently related to aggression and violence. These experiences are described below.

In reading through these experiences, it is important to remember several basic principles, as described above. First of all, multiple prenatal traumas are more likely to result in violence and aggression than single traumas. Secondly, bonding deficiencies are directly related to aggression and violence. The greater the degree of bonding deficits, the greater the likelihood of violence and aggression. Third, prenatal traumas that involve loss, abandonment or rejection are more likely to impact bonding than other traumatic themes, and are also more likely to result in the complete absence of bonding than traumas involving other themes. Finally, the direct exposure to aggression and violence during the prenatal period is highly predictive of violence and aggression during adulthood. The old adage, "Children learn what they live," is relevant here. Like children, prenates "learn what they live," and prenates subjected to aggression and violence are likely to manifest the same in their adult lives.

Conception

When clients who have problems with aggression and violence are regressed, they frequently encounter the experience of conception. They report that they are conscious of traumatic issues outside of themselves, in their family or immediate surroundings. The most frequently mentioned traumas involved forced sex, manipulated sex, date rape, rape, substance abuse, physical abuse, dismal familial, social, or cultural conditions, and personal or cultural shame, such as when children are conceived out of wedlock. They often experience biological encounters as sperm and/or eggs which involve intense aggression, annihilation, death, power, and/or rejection. To cite an example of traumatic conception, one child was conceived out of wedlock in a small religious community where such things were disdained. Her mother experienced shame, guilt, and public ridicule before deciding to "keep her," and the child experienced the same guilt, shame and ridicule that her mother did. The public ridicule was experienced as particularly annihilating and hostile. This led to character patterns of self-righteousness, self-ridicule, masochism and hostility.

Implantation

Implantation is the biological process whereby the conceptus attaches itself to the uterine wall, and is a vital and precarious stage of embryological development. Prior to and during implantation, regressed patients report that they experienced the terror of being near death. They report *feeling* unwanted and that they have no place to go, no place to belong, and 'decide' that the world is a hostile and unsafe place. They often collapse in hopelessness, retaliate in rage, fluctuate between these two extremes, and/or manifest intense rescue complexes (the need to rescue others and/or be rescued).

Vanishing Twin

Many individuals with problems of aggression report the loss of a twin. Their problems with aggression typically have to do with masochism and/or neurotic self criticism. Embryological research indicates that loss of a twin may be much more likely than previously thought. Embryologists estimate that between 30% to 80% of conceptions are actually multiple (i.e. twins) rather than single. Since the rate of birthed twins is far less than 30% to 80% percent, embryologists conclude that many conceptions involved the death of one or more twins. This is usually prior to or during implantation, although some happen after implantation.

People who experience the loss of a twin manifest several common dynamics. First of all, there is an ineffable **but** profound sense of loss, despair, and rage. These *feelings* are usually held in, **but** are sometimes acted out against others. Secondly, there is a chronic **but** unarticulated fear that loss will happen again, and pervasive insecurity. The threat of loss is defended against by distancing from others, or by engaging in codependent relationships. Third, the ability to bond with others is deficient or neurotic because there is a lack of trust in relationships, or disbelief that relationships will last. Fourth, there is often an over compliance in life, based on the unconscious *feeling* that "if I do something other than what is expected or wanted, I will die." Over-compliance feeds hostility and aggression toward others, since one is unable to take care of oneself when constantly complying with others. Finally, prenatal experiences of near death and/or loss are sometimes turned against oneself or others, resulting in sadistic and masochistic behaviors, criminal violence, or sadomasochistic thinking and behavior.

Discovery Of Unwanted Pregnancy

When aggressive clients regress to the prenatal period, they frequently and spontaneously regress to the time the pregnancy was discovered, and many of them are surprised to find that they were unwanted. The prenate's *feeling* of being unwanted can lead to lifelong episodes of depression, self-destructiveness or aggression unless the *feeling* is healed and released. The clients typically report that they can trust only themselves, and that their whole lives have been geared toward denying or finding the acceptance and love that was un-received or withheld as prenates. The percentage of aggressive clients who were unwanted at the time of discovery is quite high, and has important implications for bonding disorders. Typical responses to being unwanted are to collapse into helplessness and hopelessness, to rage at others and the world's injustice, and/or refuse to engage in life.

Prenatal Aggression

The majority of adults with problems in aggression learn that they were unwanted at the time of discovery, **but** many of them also learn that they were exposed to other forms of aggression during the prenatal and perinatal period. Some common forms of aggression are warfare, gang fights, domestic violence, conception through rape, physical or sexual abuse of parents or siblings, annihilative energies, intrauterine toxicities, and/or abortion attempts. Prenates who experience one or more of these aggressive conditions are at risk for manifesting aggression and violence, and the greater the number of conditions, the greater the likelihood of aggression and violence.

Adoption

Adoption trauma refers to a broad range of painful experiences that are common to adoption. When children are adopted, they are more likely to have experienced some level of abortion trauma - there may have been direct attempts on life, abortion plans with no attempts, or abortion ideations **but** no plans. All of these are traumatizing to varying degrees. In addition they are likely to have experienced discovery trauma (child unwanted at the time of discovery), conception trauma (child unwanted at time of conception), or psychological toxicity (child exposed to mother's annihilative or ambivalent *feelings*, or to socio-cultural shame).

Adoption trauma has many different levels. The lowest level occurs when parents want their children **but** reluctantly give them up for adoption because external circumstances dictate. A higher level occurs when children are unwanted and either or both parents seriously consider abortion. The highest level occurs when parents are unequivocally opposed to having children, when pregnancies are resented, when abortions are attempted, when children are put up for adoption and when children are fostered a number of times. At high risk for aggression are children who experience the severest levels of adoption trauma.

Prenatal And Perinatal Medical Procedures

When prenates experience severe forms of traumatization, as described above, they are also likely to perceive subsequent events in similar contexts. This is especially true when subsequent events are stressful life transitions (such as birth, adolescence, first jobs, new relationships), and/or when subsequent events are symbolically similar to traumatizing events. For example, if prenates experience prenatal violence, then they are likely to experience life transitions (such as birth) in violent ways. Freud called this process recapitulation. Among other definitions, recapitulation means that prenatal experiences shape how subsequent life experiences are perceived.

The following case is an example of a mother who had only limited prenatal traumas, **but** which nevertheless influenced her baby's perceptions and experiences of the birthing process. The mother was 28 years old, and had never attempted to conceive a child. Her own mother had had difficulty conceiving children, so she was anxious about her ability to conceive. She wanted to have a child, and in spite of being unmarried, conceived a child with her boyfriend, who was also ambivalent. They conceived after much effort, whereupon the boyfriend turned brutal and violent against the mother and her baby (it was later discovered that the boyfriend's father had been abusive to him during the prenatal period). A series of beatings occurred, after which the mother fled. She spent the remainder of her pregnancy in a distant and safe place, under conditions that were close to "ideal." She was attentive to herself, her body, and to her baby. She meditated daily and earned income from work she did at home. She had an extensive and supportive family system as well as friends, and the remainder of the pregnancy was uneventful in terms of other stresses and traumas.

She devoted time to her unborn baby every day, talking and singing to him, and doing bonding exercises. She gave birth at home, and described the birth as short and simple, with no complications. In spite of having a largely positive pregnancy and an easy birth, the early abusive experiences haunted her and her baby. In particular, her baby experienced the birth as very traumatic. (This is fairly common event, even when mothers describe births as simple and uneventful). This was evident in childhood memories of his third trimester and birth. He experienced his mother's jogging during the third trimester as abusive, saying that his head bounced painfully on his mother's pelvic bones. He experienced the perineal massages (given repeatedly during birth) as intrusive, and the contractions as abusive and violent. He was aware of his mother's physical pain, *felt* the birth was hurting her, and *felt* guilty that he was unable to protect her. In short, all of his birth *feelings* appeared to be overlays and manifestations of his unresolved abuse traumas from the first trimester. It is important to realize that, even more so than children or adults, prenates perceive and interpret life experiences in terms of past experiences. This is so because prenates have insufficient neurological integrity or adequate life experiences to assist in discerning between current and historical realities. When prenates experience abandonment, rejection, violence, or abuse, as has been described in this paper, they routinely bring these experiences to bear during the birthing process. Amniocentesis needles and chorionic villae catheters are commonly perceived as aggressive, annihilating, and/or rejecting instruments. Anesthetic procedures are often perceived as attempts to disempower or to poison (a reflection of abortion trauma). Augmentations (inductions and "breaking waters") are usually experienced as boundary violations. Forceps and vacuum extractions are often perceived as attempts to control or annihilate.

Contractions are often perceived as attempts to annihilate, destroy, or impede. For example, one adult who had been exposed to chemical and mechanical abortion attempts (his mother had taken low-dose cyanide pills and repeatedly pummeled her abdomen and uterus) experienced contractions as attempts to beat him to death, and experienced anesthesia administrations as attempts to poison him. It is vital that medical and obstetrical personnel understand the importance and relevance of prenatal and perinatal traumas, and understand that babies are likely to experience the birthing process in terms of prior traumatizations. This means that birth can be very traumatic, simply on the basis of personal history. If this fact were known, then medical interventions could be limited to situations where they were absolutely necessary, or medical interventions could be humanized in a variety of ways. Some useful procedures might be asking the permission of babies to implement procedures and getting responses through the mother's intuition, letting babies know that they might experience pains and discomforts, and empathizing in terms of prior traumas. Also, let babies know that birth is a difficult transition with the potential for negative and overwhelming *feelings* and acknowledge babies post-birth emotions as legitimate expressions of a difficult birthing process. All this could help to minimize potential trauma and heal past traumas of the prenate. It is also important to acknowledge the positive aspects of birthing; the wonder and joy that belongs to the birthing process. Few births are entirely difficult, and few are completely free from trauma or pain. We need to acknowledge the whole gamut of human experiences as they unfold during the birthing process.\

Treatment

It is important that prenatal and perinatal traumas be treated (healed) as early as possible. This is because, as previously discussed, early traumas shape how subsequent events will be perceived and experienced. If treatment occurs early on, during gestation or the first year, then childhood experiences can be freed from prenatal influences, and children can live their lives unencumbered by the bonds of trauma. The effects of trauma have been described elsewhere (Emerson, 1992, 1994). Unresolved traumas affect the spiritual and psychological development of children. In contrast, children who had no trauma, or whose traumas have been resolved, are clearly unique in the following ways. They are more spiritually evolved, manifest higher levels of human potential, and are developmentally precocious. They exhibit higher self-esteem, have higher intelligence test scores, and they are more empathic, emotionally mature, cooperative, creative, affectionate, loving, focused and self-aware than untreated and traumatized children (Emerson, 1993).

Even though prenatal and perinatal traumas shape how subsequent life events are experienced, childhood experiences, in and of themselves, are still important in terms of human development. Childhood experiences are very important in determining and shaping who children will become. It is precisely because childhood experiences are so important that it is vital to free childhood from the bonds of prenatal and perinatal trauma. If these traumas can be resolved before childhood, then childhood has the opportunity to be experienced on its own, without traumatic influence from the prenatal period, and without the defensive forces that inhibit *feelings* of safety, security and growth. Furthermore, children can be freed to exhibit and manifest their own unique human potential, to utilize their own inherent levels of intelligence and to become themselves, unencumbered by prior traumas.

In addition to these benefits, society can be freed from the increasing burden of aggression and violence. According to statistics reported at the 1995 APPPAH Congress, violence and aggression have been on the rise and reaching epidemic proportions. Therapists who specialize in anger resolution report that about one client in five carries a significant degree of anger and rage. Aggression and violence are extremely costly in terms of human lives, in terms of financial and budgetary considerations (prisons, jails, and law enforcement are very costly, and deprive our school systems of needed finances) and in terms of the safe and efficient functioning of our institutions. These violent *feelings* are directed toward self and others, and are very difficult to resolve for the following reasons. First of all, most therapists are unaware that anger and rage, at their deepest levels, are caused by prenatal and perinatal traumas, and are related to perinatal bonding deficits.

Secondly, most clinicians fail to realize that talking therapies by themselves are unable to resolve anger and rage. Instead, anger and rage require emotional healing and release. The physical release of anger in a safe and appropriate manner may also be required. Third, anger and rage are inextricably intertwined with low self-esteem, shame, guilt, disempowerment, and forgiveness. These concepts need to be understood and recognized in the treatment of aggressive disorders. Finally, the ultimate resolution of rage and anger requires that relevant prenatal and perinatal traumas be uncovered, encountered, catharted, repatterned and integrated into consciousness.

Additional aspects of treatment should include opportunities for re-bonding, i.e., for bonding in ways that were impossible at the time of traumatization, or bonding in ways that were inhibited by unresolved traumas. The Association for Prenatal and perinatal Psychology and Health, the International Primal Association, The Star Foundation, and Emerson Training Seminars have personnel and lists of professionals who do such work.

Adapted by author from <http://birthpsychology.com/free-article/vulnerable-prenate>Dec 2013

Vanishing Twins

Definition Of Vanishing Twins

Dr. Kurt Benirschke, professor of Pathology and Reproductive Medicine, states that since the advent of sonography, the number of witnessed occurrences of a fetus spontaneously vanishing is now documented. Before sonography these vanishing twins or multiple-pregnancy fetuses had been identified only occasionally. The twins were ascertained mainly when pregnancies had incidental radiography, or when placentas were examined by a pathologist. In 1989, the term "Vanishing Twin" was mentioned by Elizabeth Noble who noted that the surviving fetus experiences grief, anger and despair. She estimated that in about 4% of all pregnancies, a co-twin dies at sometime without a trace. These deeply repressed memories of loss begin to emerge in various kinds of therapies. When such memories do surface, they witness what the co-twin was *feeling* at the time of the loss. Clearly though, vanished twins have always existed and were seen much less frequently until sonography became a practical tool. Sometimes when twins are recognized by sonography, one embryo truly vanishes and is untraceable, even by skilled examination of the delivered placenta. S. Levi, who studied over 6,000 early pregnancies sonographically, found that of the 188 sets of twins identified, only 86 sets were delivered as twins. From this it was inferred that the others had "vanished." This means that there were twins **but** only a single one was born. The earlier the diagnosis of twins was made, the more frequently a twin apparently disappeared! The embryos of the dead twin may become incorporated into the placental membranes. The surviving twin may occasionally display congenital abnormalities. When one twin dies later in pregnancy and the gestation continues for some time, the water of the dead twin's tissue may be reabsorbed and the dead fetus can become flattened from pressure of the growing twin. The most widely discussed consequence of twin death is the possible occurrence of widespread damage in a surviving twin physically and emotionally. Dr David B Chamberlain, psychologist, states that the earlier a fetus or infant is subjected to pain, the greater the potential for harm. Pain makes deep impression on fetuses and babies. The younger the person the more impressionable and damaging the pain, anger, grief and loss may become.

Adapted by author from: <http://www.vanishingtwin.com/index.php/main-menu-definition> on 12/16/2013. Originally Found in 2009

The Vanishing Twin Phenomenon

In an email Mandi wrote:

"Hi,

*My name is Mandi... I am 11. A few years ago I told my mom that I had a twin, and I wanted to know where she was NOW I was kind of kidding **but** kind of serious. My mom looked at me and said "Um, yes, you had a twin...in my Stomach. **But** she died." I was shocked because she had never told me... Apparently when I was born there was two placentas, **but** just me.*

I have told only a few people about my twin (Lexie, is what I call her because that's what my mom was going to name my brother if he was a girl, and she wanted to name me that, too) Because I told my step brother once (who is a twin, too) and he called me "Baby-eater" and said I ate her...that's why I wanted to find out about Lexie.

*About the voices in the head... I do talk to myself sometimes, **but** I never thought of it much until I read your web page.*

About the genius thing...I took an online IQ test and I am 178... I am pretty sure that is genius... I am lonely a lot even with friends.

That's all I have to say.

Mandi"

An Overview By Caryl Dennis

The Vanishing Twin Phenomenon or Syndrome (VTP), as it is known in the medical literature, is explored extensively in the 1995 text *Multiple Pregnancy: Epidemiology, Gestation & Perinatal Outcome*. With contributions from over 80 experts from around the world, this book offers a definitive and comprehensive examination of the subject of twins. In it, Dr. Charles Boklage states: "In reality...losing one or both offspring from a twin pregnancy is too common to be called phenomenal, and occurs for too many different reasons to qualify as a syndrome. There is little room to doubt that the question of vanishing twins and sole survivors of twin gestation represent issues of broad and fundamental importance." With the growing use of fertility drugs and in vitro fertilization, the number of twin (or multiple) pregnancies is soaring.

From the work of Dr. Thomas Verny, Dr. David Chamberlain and others, we now know that the fetus has consciousness and memory. Dr. Verny declares in *The Secret Life of the Unborn Child*, "Birth and prenatal experiences form the foundations of human personality. Everything we become or hope to become, our relationships with ourselves, our parents, our friends, all are influenced by what happens to us in these two critical periods."

My preliminary interviews with over 200 "twinless twins" indicates that the loss of a twin in utero can have profound physical, mental and emotional effects, both on the surviving child and its parents — especially if it is unacknowledged. Unfortunately, I have found very few instances in which healthcare providers discuss these potential problems with the parents. The surviving twin may never learn of the loss of its companion; myriad psychological problems can result, with no context in which to process them. Parents are often left with unacknowledged *feelings* of confusion, loss and/or grief.

History

As early as 1945, the *Text of Obstetrics* mentioned the possibility of many more twins being conceived than born, **but** the VTP received its current name in 1980 at the Third International Congress on Twin Studies held in Jerusalem. When the subject was raised, one of the congress participants cried out, *"Vanishing twins!"* In 1995, Lawrence Wright published an extensive article, *Double Mystery*, in the New Yorker magazine which gave the VTP some public exposure.

Multiple Pregnancy: Epidemiology, Gestation & Perinatal Outcome (cited above) is the first medical text I found that addresses the VTP in great depth.

Statistics

Dr. Charles Boklage studied reports of 325 twin pregnancies and found that 61 ended as twins, 125 as singletons and the remaining 186 as a complete loss — a measure of how risky twin pregnancies are. "Somewhere in the vicinity of 10 to 15 per cent of us — that's a minimum estimate – are walking around thinking we're singletons when in fact we're only the big half", according to Boklage. He estimates that for every set of twins born alive, there are at least six singletons who are survivors of twin conceptions. Due to improved ultrasound technology and earlier detection of pregnancy, we are now able to see and document a phenomenon that has been occurring all along.

Suffering Twins

It is clear to me from my research that many surviving twins are suffering greatly from their in utero loss. It is now known that multiples interact with one another physically in the womb as early as 8 weeks into gestation. Apparently, relationships can be established very early on, the termination of which may be quite traumatic to the survivors. Due to a deep longing for some undefined, missing part of themselves that, it seems, no mate can quite fulfill, single twins may experience problems with relationships, and/or with their sexual identity. They often suffer from *feelings* of guilt. They may be haunted by *feelings* that they're "parasites". I've heard from more than a few single twins who for one reason or another *felt* they'd "eaten" or "killed" their twin. Troubling, recurring dreams of their twin, fear of sleeping alone, fear of sudden loss or abandonment, profound loneliness, eating disorders, "hearing voices", extreme emotional sensitivity and even schizophrenia or multiple personality disorder can afflict survivors of the VTP. If they are unaware that they are twinless twins, they have no context in which to place these disturbing and very confusing emotions. The good news is that, if the survivor is aware of what happened, the trauma can be processed and overcome, sometimes quite rapidly.

Elizabeth Noble says, "…unlike cases of survivor guilt from accidents, the experience of twin loss (in utero) is remembered only by the subconscious and therefore is unavailable for discussion, rationalization, and integration without assistance. It sometimes needs to be brought to the awareness of the surviving twins conscious mind for whom information about a twin's death is hidden. Those who are unaware of a vanished twin or are prohibited from expressing their *feelings* about the loss, suffer most."

Parents

The parents of VTP survivors may suffer confusion and unresolved *feelings* of great loss unless the VTP is carefully explained to them and allowances made for the grief a parent *feels* upon losing an offspring, whatever the circumstances. Unfortunately, busy doctors and our society's general attitude toward death (ignore it as much as possible on the personal level, while often obsessing about it on a cultural level) usually result in both parents and child being left in the dark.

What Are The Physical Signs For The mother Of A Possible "Vanishing Twin?"

Cramps, bleeding, and/or decreased hormone levels during the first trimester, say the doctors. Often there are no physical symptoms at all. Also, if there is a history of twins in the family and/or if a woman has already borne twins, the chances increase for VTP incidence.

Medical Opinion

Mainstream medical opinion is that these fetuses are "resorbed" by the surviving twin or the mother. Occasionally the remnants of a twin are found in the placenta or, more rarely, in a teratoma or dermoid tumor, which may contain hair, bone, teeth or other fetal tissue, and which may occur inside or outside the surviving twin or in the mother. According to a leading obstetrician I interviewed, the "resorption" explanation is only viable before the second trimester, and leaves the cases I have encountered in which the fetus disappeared as late as seven months into gestation unexplained.

Reasons For Bleeding During Pregnancy (other than the VTP):

Miscarriage: Bleeding while pregnant may indicate a pending miscarriage is certain. About half of the women who bleed have an otherwise normal pregnancy. Miscarriage can occur at any time during the first half of pregnancy. Most occur during the first 12 weeks. Miscarriage occurs in about 15 to 20 percent of pregnancies. If you think you have passed fetal tissue, take it to the doctor's office so it can be examined.

Threatened miscarriage: You may be told you are in danger of miscarrying if you experience some bleeding or cramping. The fetus is definitely still inside the uterus (based usually on an exam using ultrasound), **but** the outcome of your pregnancy is still in question. This may occur if the developing fetus is abnormal in some way, if you have an infection (of the urinary tract, for example), get dehydrated, use certain drugs or medications, suffer physical trauma… or for no apparent reason at all. There is generally another cause of miscarriage other than, or in addition to, things such as heavy lifting, exercise, having sex or emotional stress.

Incomplete miscarriage: You may have an incomplete miscarriage (or a miscarriage in progress) if the pelvic exam shows your cervix is open and you are still passing blood, clots or tissue. The cervix should remain open for only a short time. If it remains open for a long time, it indicates an incomplete miscarriage. This may occur if the uterus begins to clamp down before all the tissue has passed or if there is infection.

First trimester bleeding is, obviously enough, any vaginal bleeding during the first 3 months of pregnancy. It can vary from light spotting to severe bleeding with clots. Vaginal bleeding is a common problem in early pregnancy, complicating 20-30% of all pregnancies.

Completed miscarriage: The most common cause of first trimester bleeding is the completed miscarriage (also called spontaneous abortion). If bleeding and cramping have slowed down and the uterus appears to be empty based on ultrasound evaluation, the pregnancy can be considered terminated, the fetus lost. The causes are the same as those listed for a threatened miscarriage.

Ectopic pregnancy: Ectopic or tubal pregnancy is the most dangerous cause of first trimester bleeding. Diagnosis is based on your medical history, ultrasound, and in some cases laboratory results. An ectopic pregnancy occurs when the fertilized egg implants outside of the uterus, most often in the fallopian tube. As the fertilized egg grows, it can rupture the fallopian tube and cause life-threatening bleeding. Symptoms vary and may include pain, bleeding, or lightheadedness. Most ectopic pregnancies will cause pain before the tenth week of pregnancy. The fetus instead of developing, will die because it lacks a supply of nutrients. This condition occurs in about 3% of all pregnancies. Risk factors for ectopic pregnancy include a history of prior ectopic pregnancy, history of pelvic inflammatory disease, history of fallopian tube surgery or ligation, history of infertility for more than two years, having an IUD (birth control device placed in the uterus) in place, smoking, or frequent (daily) douching. Only about 50% of women who experience an ectopic pregnancy have any risk factors, however.

Implantation bleeding: There can be a small amount of spotting associated with the normal implantation of the embryo into the uterine wall, called implantation bleeding. This is usually very minimal, **but** frequently occurs on or about the same day as the menstrual period is due, which can result in its being mistaken for a mild menstrual discharge and the mistaken belief that there is no pregnancy. Implantation bleeding is a normal part of pregnancy and no cause for concern.

Blighted ovum (embryonic failure): Although an ultrasound shows evidence of an intrauterine pregnancy, the embryo fails to develop as it should, most likely due to abnormalities in the fetus itself, as opposed to something the mother did or failed to do.

Intrauterine fetal demise (IUFD — also called missed abortion, or embryonic demise): The developing baby dies inside the uterus, for any of the same reasons a threatened miscarriage occurs during the early stages of pregnancy. This diagnosis would be based on ultrasound results and can occur at any time during pregnancy, although it is rare in the second and third trimesters. Causes also include separation of the placenta from the uterine wall (called placental abruption) and insufficient blood flow into the placenta.

Molar pregnancy (technically known as gestational trophoblastic disease): Ultrasound may reveal that the presumed developing fetus is actually abnormal tissue. This is actually a type of cancer that occurs as a result of the hormones of pregnancy. In rare cases the abnormal tissue invades the uterine wall and metastasizes, thereby threatening the life of the mother.

Postcoital bleeding is vaginal bleeding after sexual intercourse while pregnant. It is common within limits.

Higher Risk

Twins and higher-order multiples appear to be at greater risk of neurological and cognitive problems than singletons, as well as a vast array of physical problems. To name **but** a few: malformations of the cardiovascular, gastrointestinal and central nervous systems, kidney and organ misplacement, auto-immune disorders, clubfoot, extra fingers or toes. Also, current studies are confirming a previously suspected link between cerebral palsy and the twinning process. There are many websites available with information on this connection.

Chimera

A curious phenomenon of the twinning process is the chimera, an individual with different cell populations derived from more than one fertilized egg. According to Lawrence Wright's *Double Mystery* article, "Charles Boklage cites (speaking of the chimera)…though it has rarely been detected, it may be more common than it seems. 'Possibly some of us are twins who are walking around in a single body,' Boklage says…Occasionally, blood donors are found to be carrying two different blood types: it could mean that fraternal twins merged in the womb. Of course, there is no way to determine whether identical twins have merged, since their genes and blood types are the same. In those cases, the twins amalgamate (combine into one) instead of vanishing."

After I gave a talk on the VTP, a woman came up to me and said, "Now I know what's happening to my husband. This explains it!" She told me that her husband was occasionally "different, somehow" — he looked the same, **but** there was something wrong. It was most apparent to her when they made love. One day she asked him if he really was her husband, and he replied imperiously, in a loud, flat voice: "We will **not** speak of that again!" It frightened the woman to the extent that she never did. She told me, "They're switching him. Now I know for sure." According to his mother, this fellow was a VTP survivor.

Ethical Issues

The increased use of fertility procedures is presenting doctors and potential parents with new moral and ethical problems. Because an infertile couple spends between $1,500 and $6,000 per attempt, there is a tendency for doctors to place multiple fertilized eggs, often resulting in multiple viable fetuses. Because of the greater odds against bringing multiples successfully to term, doctors may resort to a procedure known as multifetal pregnancy reduction (MFPR) in order to increase the probability of producing at least one healthy child. This of course places parents in the difficult position of deciding whether to abort one or more of the new lives they have struggled (and paid dearly!) to start. MFPR may also place the entire pregnancy in danger (although risks are being reduced with practice). The trauma of the procedure may itself create devastating psychological problems for the prenate, just as an attempted abortion that unknowingly takes only one of a set of twins can mentally and emotionally scar the survivor, leaving him or her with the same psychological issues as a twinless twin.

DES (a drug)

Between the early 1940's and 1971, a drug called Diethylstilbestrol (DES) was given as a miscarriage prevention measure to between 5 and 10 million pregnant women who were, usually, bleeding vaginally. Bleeding during pregnancy is known to be a sign of the VTP, when there are any signs at all. It is also known that twinning rates increase after a period of sexual abstinence.

The post-World War II "baby boom" came after just such a period. I suspect that many of the women given DES at that time were experiencing the VTP — hence the bleeding.

Sonographers

A number of sonographers at a convention I attended in 1996 expressed frustration about a situation that apparently occurs too often: early in her pregnancy, a mother receives a sonogram. The sonographer and/or the doctor spot two fetuses. Subsequently, however, one "vanishes". By way of explanation, the busy doctor may tell the mother that the sonographer made a mistake or merely dismiss the whole thing with a remark like, "It happens all the time. Be glad you're only having one!" Imagine the sonographer's frustration. Potential psychological issues of the prenate are left unaddressed.

Psychological Help

NET

Scott Walker, D.C., (a twinless twin) has developed a process of psychological kinesiology and spinal adjustments known as Neuro-Emotional Technique (NET), which he has taught to thousands of chiropractors. Dr. Walker incorporates information on the VTP into his training; many people are discovering their twinship through the NET process. I have communicated with many of these people, as well as some of the chiropractors, and found that a desire for more clear, accessible information about the VTP is widespread.

Psychic Bond

There is certainly no shortage of anecdotal evidence of the existence of psychic bonds between twins. The "Jim twins", identicals who were separated at birth and raised apart, made sensational headlines when they eventually found each other. Both had been named Jim, both had married a woman named Linda and subsequently divorced her. Both remarried, this time to women named Betty. One twin named his first son James Alan, the other James Allan; both had owned a dog named Toy; both worked part-time as deputy sheriffs; both had been employed by McDonald's and both had been attendants in filling stations. Both spent their holidays at St. Petersburg Beach, FL, and both drove Chevrolets to get there. Both bite their fingernails and drink Miller Lite Beer. Both built a white bench around the trunk of a tree in their respective gardens. These are **but** some of the astonishing parallels in their separate lives.

One has only to attend a "Twinless Twin" conference and hear the attendees tell of knowing when their twin died, of *feeling* their pain and of communicating with them after death to see that there is something unique — beyond coincidence — about the bonds between twins, and that it may continue even with the death of one of them.

Some people believe that there is no evidence that twins' similarities are caused by mental communication between them. Perhaps this is because it is difficult to obtain grant funds to thoroughly research such things, or perhaps it is because the clinical research setting disturbs the psychic process in some way.

Personal Experience

I began researching the VTP in 1993 after finding out that I am a surviving twin and that my fraternal twin siblings probably began as triplets, and that my youngest brother was a surviving "mirror" identical twin. I also have a cousin who is a "mirror" identical twin (her twin vanished), whose organs are on the opposite side of her body. My mother took DES during my pregnancy. I have traveled extensively since 1993, researching and lecturing to hundreds of people on the VTP. I've heard many fascinating and often heart-breaking stories. My web site, which generates emails from surviving twins from around the world, has been up since 1997. Numerous guest appearances on national radio and TV programs have also generated a good deal of correspondence from "twinless twins" and their caregivers, as well as health and educational professionals.

In 1997 I published, with my partner Parker Whitman, *The Millennium Children: Tales of the Shift.* This book contains a large section on the VTP, along with my life story (I share much of my personal story of the discovery of my twin, who I named "Karyl") and a great deal of material concerning the increasing number of children being born today with exceptional intuitive, intellectual and physical abilities — children who speak of past lives, of "being in spirit", of "imaginary friends", and of extraterrestrial contact. Much of the information on the *Millennium Children* was gathered in the course of my research into the VTP. The *Millennium Children* has generated additional correspondence from twinless twins.

Summary

While medical information about the VTP is now available, information concerning its psychological impact is only available in bits and pieces in various publications. Dr. Nancy L. Segal, one of the nation's premiere twin researchers, states in her book *Entwined Lives: Twins and What they Tell Us about Human Behavior* (1999), "No one has systematically studied the psychological effects on children of losing a twin before birth or in infancy." VTP survivors and their parents need such information; healthcare practitioners need the knowledge and the resources to provide it. I hope that my efforts will help to address these needs.

Adapted by author from <http://caryl.ipower.com/wordpress/vanishing-twins/>

Chapter 12

Five Methods of Healing, Clearing and Releasing

Whatever method you choose of clearing, healing and releasing has four basic parts:

1) Seeing what needs to be released

2) Releasing it.

3) Cleaning up and fully relinquishing and detaching from it.

4) Filling yourself with divine light, color, love frequencies to fill up the empty places created by the release.

You have to clean up after yourself. You must process the loss. That's a rule like gravity. That's how it works. Every step in the process of awakening has all four components.

Below is adapted from *Spiritual Warfare* by Jed McKenna.

The power of the mind, the power to see clearly is the key.

As Jed's client says:

"Great! My attic is haunted! My mind is haunted. My thoughts are haunted. *I* am haunted; possessed, plagued with 'demons'. My mother is here. My unborn children are here. My future is here, my dreams. Everyone who means anything to me, good or bad, pleasant or unpleasant, is here. How do they all fit? How could I have **not** seen them right away? Of *course* they're here. *This* is where they are. My attic is me, there is no place else.

Whether or **not** they have physical counterparts out in the real world is meaningless to me, just as the fact that I might be a real person in the real world is meaningless to them. Perception is reality. I am possessed by my own perceptions; **not** by things and people, future and past, **but** by my perceptions of them. These are my connections, my attachments. Maybe all I really am is the sum of all these connections, these fearful longings and graspings. What is an attachment anyway? It's a belief, that's all. A strong one maybe, **but** just a belief. And no belief is true."

Yes, I will do away with these people inhabiting my mind. I will release and relinquish them by clearly seeing the attachments that keep them here. I can see those attachments now. I can see the emotions at work and I am starting to see them for what they are. I am starting to understand what stuff this prison of self is really made of.

I do**n't** seem to think about anything anymore. I ca**n't** even think of anything that needs thinking about. Sometimes I try to think about something, latch onto something and give it some thought, **but** it just fades after a moment or two. Thought for me is a tool, a weapon. The only reason to lug it out is if something needs to be released and detached. It's a sword, **but** I have nothing left to swing it at. I pick it up desultorily and cleave the air, **but** it's just the empty reminiscences of an old soldier. What would I think about? Religion? Politics? Business? The arts? I am blank. I am, by Emerson's reckoning, nothing.

My general state most closely resembles a kind of bittersweet gladness. I do**n't** dwell in my memories, I'm **not** even sure if I really have any. It seems like I have a box of old movie footage somewhere in my mental space, **but** the idea of hauling it out and reminiscing over the clumsily spliced scenes of a life with which I feel no connection holds no appeal. I know that I was once a warrior, **but** it's **not** the memory of that state of being, just the recollection of a fact. There's no pleasure or displeasure in it. It's like something you know about someone else. McKenna, Jed. (2007). *Spiritual Warfare.* (p. 212-213)

Yogi Berra(a professional baseball player) said, "If the world were perfect, it would**n't** be." (1947 in St Louis)

We can do our best to stay as true as we can to our mission and principles

If we were born in utopia, would it be perfect? Life is a journey. To appreciate the sunrise we must first pass through the night. How can we truly understand happiness and health without pain and sickness? Being born perfect would be nice, **but** attaining perfection by one's own will sounds like the trip of a lifetime. What do you think? Would a perfect world be perfect?

There is a place where all paradoxes disappear and where no questions remain. Once you are there you will know. There is no point in trying to describe this place.

Practices For Healing, Transmuting, Releasing And Integrating

Prayer Practice

Prayer is basically a sincere attempt to communicate with and to Source and the Divine within yourself. The key is to be present, authentic and sincere with LOVE in your heart. Practice your own prayers instead of repeating other's words from memory. True prayer comes from the heart. Words (spoken or silent) only start and guide prayer.

Affirmations Practice

Affirmations are often described as positive statements. They are used to retrain the Unihipili (subconscious mind) and create constructive changes in yourself and the physical world.

Every thought and word is an affirmation. All of our inner dialogues are streams of affirmations. Saying and thinking positive affirmations will help to shift you from the negative to the positive. Each negative thought and word will create more of the negative. Affirmations function at the level of the Unihipili (subconscious mind) and are very powerful. Avoiding the use of the words *not, but, need to, try, want to, should* and *could* is critical in affirmations. Realize *don't, won't, can't, shouldn't* are all "not" words.

The Universe only understands Truth (yes). It is critical to use the positive counterpart of any negative. If you find yourself thinking or saying something negative or unkind say to yourself and the universe, "cancel/clear", and rethink or reword with something positive and kind.

If you say, "I will not be Angry" or "I am not angry", the Universe hears, "I will be angry" or "I am angry".

Instead say, "I will be forgiving, LOVING" or "I am forgiving, LOVING" (unconditional love).

If you have difficulty thinking of an appropriate word, use the positive word or words that come the closest.

Interestingly, when you think or say, "I am not happy", the universe keeps the 'not' in place and energizes the opposite of happy. Be mindful of how you think and speak.

If there are negative and/or limiting *feelings*, emotions, memories or beliefs involved, the effectiveness of positive affirmations <u>may</u> be limited until the *feelings*, emotions, memories replaying or beliefs involved are healed, transmuted, released and integrated. Sometimes the affirmation itself creates the healing.

At first, it may be difficult for you to avoid using the thoughts or words *not, try, need to, should*. It gets easier with practice. In normal daily conversation and occasionally when doing healing, I still catch myself using negative or limiting words and phrases. Thinking positive thoughts, saying positive words and re-wording your thoughts and statements will become easier with practice, forgiveness and LOVE.

Memories Replaying Practice
Erasing The Energetic Attachment To And *Feelings* From 'Memories Replaying'

Memories replaying are like old tapes from past experiences that keep negative and limiting beliefs energized. For example, one might delete an email. However, until the 'deleted' folder is emptied and the email is permanently trashed the email is still there and so is the message.

Ho'oponopono is an ancient Hawaiian method of healing and clearing. A good introduction to Self I-dentity through Ho'oponopono, as taught by Ihaleakala Hew Len, is the book, *Zero Limits*, by Joe Vitale and Ihaleakala Hew Len. Self I-dentity Ho'oponopono has been overly commercialized, by some. However, if you get beyond the greed and loss of integrity, by some, and to the original Self I-dentity through Ho'oponopono, as taught by Ihaleakala Hew Len, you will find it a valuable tool for healing and clearing.

Sometimes the following method is taught as, "I Love you. I am sorry. Please forgive me. Thank you." I *feel* that as you progress it may be best to say, "I Love you. Thank you," with the awareness that at the level of Spirit there is nothing to be sorry for or to be forgiven. Say it with sincerity, whichever ways *feels* best to you at the time. Remember that all sources of hurt and pain we have agreed to host manifest as internal self-agreements. Say the following statements mentally. There is no need to project them to the person or situation that hurt, mistreated or angered you. If you feel someone is unforgivable, say them anyway with no thought of the person. Only say them out loud if clearly guided.

"I LOVE You"
  Said to "All That Is" and to whomever or whatever has upset you, hurt you, made you sad, made you fearful, even if you have no idea why you are fearful, sad, angry, or judgmental.

"Thank You"
  Said to "All That Is" and whomever or whatever has upset you, hurt you, made you sad, made you fearful, even if you have no idea why your upset.

  You are thankful for the opportunity to practice "Unconditional Divine LOVE" and heal and clear whatever is of something other than LOVE.

"Clean and Erase as is best"
  You are healing, transmuting, releasing and erasing the memory replaying that has energized hurt, sadness, attack or anger. The actual memory may remain, however the energy attached to the memory will be healed, transmuted and released and will no longer affect you. This also often heals, transmutes and releases the 'negative', and integrates the positive counterpart of any associated trapped or suppressed *feelings*/emotions. There are many memories replaying and energizing hurts and beliefs, so realize this is an ongoing practice.

Adapted from *Zero Limits* by Ihaleakala Hew Len and Joe Vitale (p. 30-32) and from a seminar on Self I-dentity through Ho'oponopono given by Hew Len in 2009.

It is vital that we understand what *really* was or still is affecting us. It was or still is our own beliefs, decisions, agreements and behaviors that manifest our realities.

Releasing Trapped Feelings and Emotions Practice

The information in this section is based on Dr. Bradley Nelson's book, *The Emotion Code* and was excerpted from his website in 2009. The web page is no longer available. His current web site is <http://www.drbradleynelson.com/> as of February 14, 2014.

Explanation of "The Emotion Code" by Dr. Bradley Nelson – August 31, 2007

In the battle for primacy in healing and wellness, will the medical communities' pharmaceutical/ surgical approach prevail, or will Western Medicine as we know it become a team player in a more enlightened, more integrated approach?

There is tremendous momentum at this point in the world of healing, momentum that is swinging the pendulum toward a more natural approach to health. As a practicing holistic chiropractic physician for nearly 20 years now, I have learned a few things about this topic that you might be surprised to learn. I have developed my own method of healing, the BodyCode, which has enabled me to heal many otherwise incurable patients, all without drugs or surgical intervention.

First, one of my favorite quotes by Thomas Edison. He said, "The doctor of the future will give no medicine, **but** will interest his patients in the care of the human frame, in diet, and in the cause and prevention of disease," and while we may have yet to arrive at this state of affairs regarding the health care system in America quite yet, I do believe we are moving in that general direction.

To let you know a little more about me, I have recently published a book called "The Emotion Code," and I regularly speak and lecture nationally via both TV and radio on alternative health care methods, particularly regarding the emotional aspect of disease. I have successfully treated and corrected a wide variety of ailments including ADD, ADHD, asthma, allergies, back pain, Bell's palsy, carpal tunnel syndrome, chronic fatigue syndrome, depression, fibromyalgia, headaches, herniated discs, hiatal hernia, hip pain, infertility, lack of energy, knee pain, learning disabilities, lupus, migraines, neck pain, shoulder pain, sinus problems and vertigo, all with natural methods, without drugs and without surgery.

If you will bear with me, I will teach you what I believe to be the underlying causes of all sickness and disease. I will also explain how these causes can be corrected and health can be restored naturally without drugs.

First of all let's take a look at traditional medicine. Western Medicine as we know it was born in the civil wars and during the world wars, and developed around a concept that I call 'heroic measures.' What does that mean? It means that if a cannonball comes bouncing along the field and takes off your leg, your doctor will perform life-saving procedures, stopping your blood loss and saving your life. There are times when 'heroic measures' are entirely appropriate. There were many good and heroic doctors in those wars, just as there continues to be now.

Unfortunately, we have come to base our whole health care system around heroic measures. In spite of all the talk about preventive medicine, we still wait until there is a crisis before we act. As a result, Western Medicine focuses on external causes of disease, on dramatic interventions such as organ transplants, and on symptom suppression. Of course, symptom suppression is performed with pharmaceutical drugs. Drugs unfortunately are now the third leading cause of death in the country. We spend more money on health care than any other country on earth per capita, and yet we now rank among the least healthy countries in the world, recently ranking 47th in overall health.

When you rely on drugs to suppress symptoms, things can really start to go wrong. To give you an idea what can happen, let's take a look at a cartoon by Klaber and Gongoll called "The Last Alternative", "Side Effects", or "Who Says the Medical System has major problems?"

Susie went to her doctor with a cough. He prescribed the antibiotic Amoxicillin and said, "This will take care of it." As a side effect of the antibiotic, Susie gets a yeast infection, so her doctor prescribes the anti fungal drug Diflucan and says, "This will take care of it." With her immune system depressed, Susie gets depressed, and her doctor prescribes the antidepressant Prozac, and says, "This will take care of it." Like it does for others, the Prozac elevates Susie's blood pressure, so her doctor prescribes the anti high-blood pressure drug Captopril and says, "This will take care of it." As is fairly common, Captopril gave Susie a cough, so her doctor prescribed the antibiotic Amoxicillin and said, "This will take care of it." And around and around we go. This sort of scenario actually happens to people, and this is the kind of thing that can occur when you are chasing symptoms and suppressing them. What's really tragic is that Susie *felt* lousy **but** lucky, because her insurance paid for 90% for all these drugs. This is the twisted reality in America today. Who is the victim here? Susie, of course. **But** her doctors are also victims of a pharmaceutical/industrial complex that is drunk with power and money, accountable to no-one.

To understand how disease occurs, it is critical that we talk about stress. Most people are intuitively aware that stress has an effect on the immune system, since a cold or an outbreak of cold sores often follows stressful episodes for many.

Noble prize nominee Dr. Hans Selye found that health is like a 'rubber band.' Stress stretches the 'rubber band' of your health, sometimes to its very limit. According to Dr. Selye, stresses include things like pregnancy, infections, surgeries, traumas, allergic reactions, immune reactions, severe exertions, strong emotions, poor diet, and severe exposures. Stresses like these will 'stretch' the 'rubber band' of your health and put your body into a state of strain.

Usually you are able to deal with the stress. You overcome the stress, shrug it off and your body returns to normal, **but** sometimes stresses are prolonged and cumulative, and the stress can overwhelm your body.

Imagine that you are walking alone in the forest when suddenly you are confronted with a grizzly bear which rears up on its hind legs and roars at you.

Your adrenal glands instantly go into action. These glands, which sit atop each kidney, are responsible for producing stress hormone such as adrenaline and cortisol. These hormones have very precise and interesting effects on the body.

First of all, they help to reroute blood away from the digestive organs and toward the skeletal muscles, so that you can either run away from the bear or fight the bear more effectively, whichever you choose to do. After all, there is no need to be digesting your lunch right now, since you could be dead in moments.

In addition, these hormones suppress the immune system. Who needs an immune system at a time like this anyway? They also release stored sugars and fats into the bloodstream so that they can be readily used as fuel in this imminent life or death struggle.

In the short-term, these are all very appropriate things for the body to do. And you might be wondering what they have to do with you and your health. After all, there are no bears in your life. Or are there? How about that stressful situation at work yesterday? How about your marriage, your kids, your aging parents? All of these things are stresses, and your body unable to tell the difference between these stresses and facing a bear. The same chemicals are released, circulating in your blood and bathing your tissues for up to 48 hours after one stressful episode.

Too many stressful episodes can 'snap' the 'rubber band' of your health. Once this occurs, like an airplane in a tailspin, you are spiraling down toward disease.

Stress has now opened the door to illness. The body's defenses are down. A whole variety of things now start to go wrong. Infections which used to be easily defeated now can become chronic. Parasites may set up permanent residence in the body as well. Because the immune system is now too weak to eliminate and destroy these invaders, it allows them to stay in your body, like unwelcome relatives who came for a visit and have now moved in permanently. Toxins also begin to accumulate in the body tissues and take their own toll on health. Allergies, misalignments of the vertebrae and other bones, energetic imbalances, and nutritional deficiencies also increase, as do trapped emotions. The body is now in a state of distortion. A remarkable characteristic of this condition is that it is rarely recognized for the perilous state that it is. In a state of distortion, your health is now being lost on daily basis.

If this situation is left in place, the inevitable end result is disease.

And what is a disease? ***Nothing more than a collection of symptoms***.

In my work with chronically ill patients, I found that there was usually no single smoking gun, no single cause of their illness. Instead, my patients all seemed to have one thing in common: they were all imbalanced in the ways that I have been describing.

Stress at some point in the past 'snapped' the 'rubber band' of their health. Their immune system became depressed. They developed energetic, structural, and chemical imbalances and their bodies began manifesting symptoms. It is my belief that all diseases occur in the same way, whether the disease is fibromyalgia, chronic fatigue, lupus, asthma, cancer, or whatever disease you can think of, with few exceptions.

It was common for my chronically ill patients to have low grade infections, parasites, nutritional deficiencies, structural misalignments, trapped emotions, and so on. All of these imbalances had to be corrected for health to return. If the individual imbalances are corrected, the body can heal itself.

Six Kinds Of Imbalance - Basic Explanation

While imbalance in general is what causes us to lose our health, we can break it down into six specific kinds of imbalance.

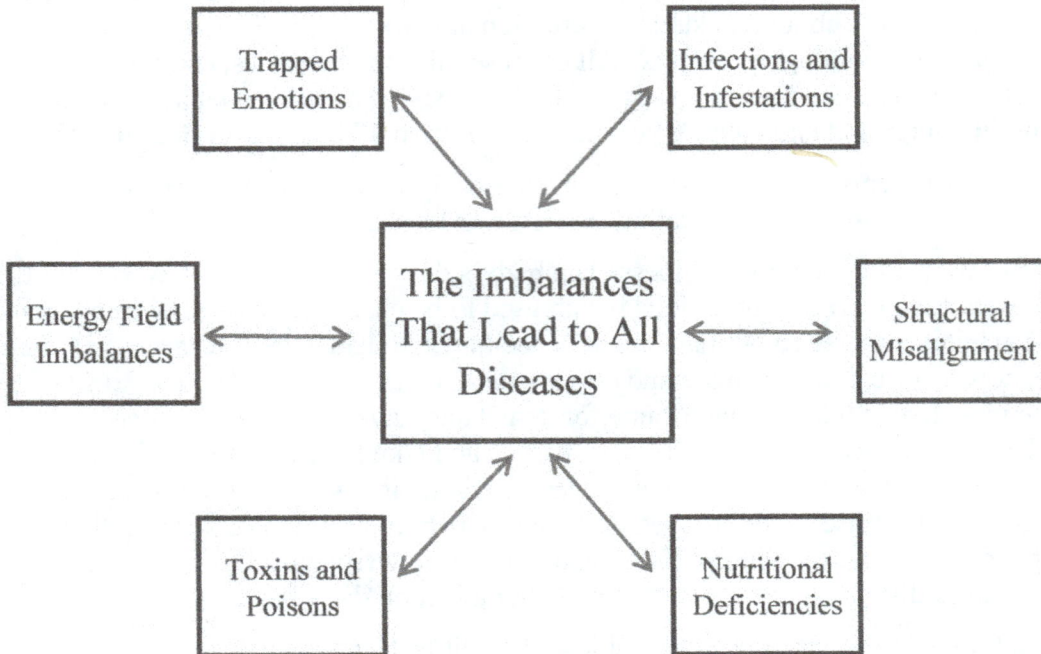

```
┌──────────────┐                    ┌──────────────┐
│   Trapped    │                    │ Infections and│
│   Emotions   │                    │  Infestations │
└──────────────┘                    └──────────────┘

┌──────────────┐    ┌──────────────────┐    ┌──────────────┐
│ Energy Field │    │  The Imbalances  │    │  Structural  │
│  Imbalances  │◄──►│ That Lead to All │◄──►│ Misalignment │
└──────────────┘    │     Diseases     │    └──────────────┘
                    └──────────────────┘

┌──────────────┐                    ┌──────────────┐
│  Toxins and  │                    │  Nutritional │
│   Poisons    │                    │ Deficiencies │
└──────────────┘                    └──────────────┘
```

The image above represents the "big picture." All disease, no matter what it might be called, is caused by the six different kinds of imbalance that you see above. It's that simple.

In a few more minutes, we will take a look at each of these imbalances more specifically, **but** for now let's talk about how we get information out of the body.

Imagine that you are bush-man living in the outback. You have never seen a car, never seen a bicycle and you have no concept of what electricity means. Now, imagine that you are presented with a modern computer. You would obviously have no clue how to even get it started, let alone make it into a productive tool. Our bodies are a bit like this. We have had them now for thousands of years **but** since they came with no manual, we have spent much of our time trying to figure out how they work and how to make them work better.

In medieval times, people thought that illness was caused by, among other things, too much blood. As a result, blood-letting was a popular practice for quite some time, until it was finally discarded.

Medical practices once thought to be good medicine are routinely abandoned as more knowledge is gained. For example, when I was a child, many of my friends had their tonsils removed at the slightest hint of trouble. The tonsils were considered expendable, and were thought to have no function at all. Now, we know that they form part of the body's immune defense, and are more important than once thought.

In our day, rather than using blood-letting, we tend to poison our bodies with toxic drugs that gradually destroy our liver and kidneys. Medications can certainly be appropriate at times, **but** are vastly over-utilized in our society. Actually, the body itself contains the answers to all that ails it.

The body has an innate ability to tell the difference between what is true and what is false. For example, if you are hooked up to a lie detector, you may tell a lie with your lips, and you might sound very convincing, **but** the polygraph machine will pick up your body's subtle imbalances and the truth will come out.

The Subconscious Mind

The subconscious mind has a built-in ability to tell the difference between what is true and what is other than truth. How much of your brain do you actually use? Probably about 10%, if you are like most people. It is said that Einstein used about 15% of his brain.

So what is the rest of your brain doing? Actually, it is cataloging and archiving everything you do in your life. Every face you have ever seen in a crowd, everything you have ever touched, tasted, smelled, every thought, every infection you have ever had, every immune defense that your body ever had to mount, is all recorded and stored as memory in the Unihipili (subconscious mind). The whole history of your health or illness is in the Unihipili (subconscious mind).

We know that the human body is essentially a binary computer, **but** how can we access that information? Starting with work on applied kinesiology or muscle testing, I have developed a method I call the Body Code, that allows us to access the information that is in the Unihipili (subconscious mind).

I believe there is a subconscious list of the exact things in the Unihipili (subconscious mind) that need to be done to get well; this information is accessed through muscle testing, whereby a weak muscle signifies a negative answer, while a strong muscle signifies a positive answer. In essence we talk to the Unihipili (subconscious mind) through the body, and the body answers.

> Glenn's note: I believe the Unihipili (subconscious mind) needs to be consciously loved and thanked for any form of knowing/asking/affirming to be truly accurate. Make sure your Unihipili (subconscious mind) is happy, loved and appreciated.

> Dr. Nelson only mentions the "Sway Test". I suggest other methods below that may be better for some people

> There are several ways to get answers from your own Unihipili (subconscious mind).

> 1) The "Sway Test"
> 2) Muscle Testing
>   a) Using the arm of a second person
>   b) Several methods you can do yourself without a second person
> 3) Using a pendulum or dowsing rods
> 4) Getting a 'Yes' or 'No' on a mental chalk board
> 5) Best of all: have a *feeling*.

Keep Your Mind Clear, Dr. Nelson (Continued)

Make sure you keep your mind clear of other thoughts after making your statement. If your thoughts are wandering, it will be difficult for your Unihipili (subconscious mind) to determine exactly what it is you are after. What if, for example, you make a positive or true statement, **but** then immediately begin thinking about the argument you had with your spouse last night? The memory of that event is negative, and your Unihipili (subconscious mind) will be confused.

It is important to have patience with yourself. When you are first learning to get answers from your Unihipili (subconscious mind) you will need to practice and persevere. Let go of any discouragement that may creep in.

Your Unihipili (subconscious mind) response time will shorten significantly the more you practice. The most challenging aspect of any form of testing for many people is that it requires them to give up control for a few moments, and allow their Unihipili (subconscious mind) the freedom to answer. For some, giving up control is difficult. Nevertheless, this is a simple skill and should take a short time to learn and to become proficient.

Next, Let's Talk About The Energy Field Within All Living Things.

Discovered in 1939 in the Ukraine, Kirlian photography allows us to view the inner energetic field of living things. All living things exhibit this same energy field, without exception.

In this picture, we can see the energy field extending out around the finger tips of the human being. This energy field is invisible to the naked eye, **but** under Kirlian photography it becomes visible. This energy field exists in all living things and is within us. If this part of us, this hidden unseen part of us, becomes imbalanced, then it becomes difficult for us to regain our health, unless it is rebalanced

My favorite Kirlian photograph was taken by a scientist in Sweden.

They took a living leaf and cut it in two. They threw the top half of the leaf away, then made a Kirlian photograph of the remaining bottom half of the leaf.

The resulting Kirlian photograph shows both the bottom half of the leaf which was physically present and the top half of the leaf which had been discarded. This same energy field exists within us and within all living things. In our bodies, if this energy field becomes imbalanced it must be rebalanced or brought back into a state of balance for us to regain our health.

Six Different Kinds Of Imbalance In Detail

As I mentioned before, there are six different kinds of imbalance that make us lose our health. Let's take a look at this in detail.

Infections And Infestations Is The First Type Of Imbalance.

Infections refers to low-grade infections which can linger in the body for years. These can be difficult or impossible to pick up on a blood test, yet they can greatly contribute to illness, loss of energy and pain. Infections may be viral such as theEpstein-barr virus, flus or colds. They can be bacterial, such as strep or staph infections, or they may be fungal, such as candidiasis, or mold. These can usually be helped and healed often without having to resort to toxic drugs.

Infestations refers to parasites. What are parasites? Parasites are small organisms often microscopic which infest your body and contribute to a loss of health. Worldwide, parasites and infections are the number one cause of death, killing over 12 million people annually. In the United States, approximately 85% of the population is infested with parasites at present. Parasites are very difficult to pick up on medical tests. Parasites can spread throughout the body causing muscle pain, joint pain, and a variety of other symptoms, and in my experience, are best dealt with through the use of specific herbal combinations.

Structural Misalignment Is The Second Type Of Imbalance.

> Glenns' note: Many people are aware of structural misalignment of the spine and see chiropractors. There is another type of structural misalignment few people are aware of. This is misalignment of the teeth and improper growth of the jaw caused by poor nutrition or injury when a person is young or even before birth. It can cause major energy blockages and lock up the 'breathing' of the cranium.

The most basic communication system in the body consists of the brain and its network of nerves. The central nervous system consists of over 1 trillion nerves cells, or neurons, which connect and control all of the cells and tissues of the body. Information from the brain travels down the spinal cord and out along various spinal nerves to all body tissues.

Let's zoom in on a section of the spine and take a closer look.

The bones that make up the spine house and protect the spinal cord. In between each vertebra, there is a hole about the size of the pencil where the nerves exit as they branch off of the spinal cord. In the neck, these nerves may travel down the arms. Nerves branching out in the upper back may go to the lungs or heart. Nerves branching out from the mid-back may go to the Stomach, and so on.

These nerves are quite tough and durable in most parts of the body, however, at the point where the nerves pass between the vertebrae, they are quite delicate. Unfortunately, sometimes vertebrae become misaligned and pressure occurs on these exiting nerves. This pressure, although slight, is often enough to cause interference in the transmission of nerve impulses. If this condition persists, then the body becomes weakened, and illness or disease can be the result.

We refer to these misalignments of the vertebrae as subluxations. Subluxations of vertebrae in the cervical spine are related to headaches, subluxations in the lower back to low back discomfort and so on. Most people have one or more subluxations. As a result, their health is endangered, and they probably unaware of it.

Misalignments may be caused by birth trauma, childhood falls and traumas, sports injuries, whiplash, excess sitting, poor diet, occupational hazards, lack of exercise, and even emotional stress. Unfortunately, sometimes there is noticeable discomfort or symptom at first from subluxations. The damage that they cause is often imperceptible in the beginning. By the way, other bones in addition to the vertebrae can become misaligned. Other tissues may need realigning in your body such as ligaments, tendons, muscles, and even internal organs, which can also become misaligned and create structural or physical imbalance.

Any misaligned tissue will usually cause pain and will always cause decreased function in the body. For example, If a vertebrae becomes misaligned in the upper back, it may interfere with the communication linkage between the brain and the lungs, the brain and the heart, and so on. Let's use the lungs as an example.

Let's suppose that you have a misalignment in the spine, creating interference in the nerves that are carrying information from the brain to the lungs. If the lungs are getting less than100% communication from the brain, will they be able to function at 100%?

The answer is logically no, and in fact, the lungs will usually begin to malfunction if this condition is left uncorrected. The body may become more prone to lung infections, may develop shortness of breath, even asthma. In fact, I have seen many cases of asthma over the years were helped and often completely eliminated simply by taking the pressure off of the nervous system.

If a vertebrae a little further down becomes misaligned what happens? Interference may develop between the brain and the gallbladder. The gallbladder helps us to digest fat, and so, indigestion will be the result, including gas and bloating. If this is allowed to continue, it may contribute to gallstones and eventual removal of the gallbladder.

If a misalignment occurs in the area of the back where the nerves are carrying information between the brain and the liver, the liver will be unable to function at peak efficiency and so the body will no longer be able to detoxify itself as well as it should. This will contribute to a toxic situation which can end up being a primary cause of fibromyalgia, chronic fatigue syndrome, loss of energy, and a variety of other problems.

If a misalignment occurs in the spine, in the area where nerves are leaving the spine and are carrying information between the brain and the uterus for example, it will be very difficult to conceive, infertility, and dysmenorrhea may be the result. By simply restoring the communication linkage between the brain and the uterus, it is possible sometimes to restore fertility if all other factors are balanced as well.

Nutritional Deficiencies Is The Third Type Of Imbalance.

Nutritional deficiency or imbalance is certainly a large factor in loss of health.

Most of the food we buy at the store is very low in nutrient quality. Researchers at Rutgers University, intrigued by the emphatic claim that "Organic is Better," decided to shop around for some answers. They went to a supermarket and purchased a selection of produce, which they analyzed for mineral content. They then went to a health food store featuring organically grown produce and repeated their purchase. The organic produce was put through the same testing. The Rutgers team expected the organic produce to be slightly superior in this comparison, **but** the results were astounding! Incredibly, many essential elements are completely absent in commercial produce. Almost every patient I saw was nutritionally deficient in some way or another. Luckily, the body knows what it needs to become balanced again, in the form of vitamins or minerals, glandular preparations, herbals, homeopathic remedies, and so on.

We have now looked at three different kinds of imbalance; Infections/infestations, structural misalignments, and nutritional deficiencies.

Toxins and Poisons Is The Fourth Type Of Imbalance.

Toxicity is the problem of the modern era. It is said that we get more toxic exposure just filling up our car with gasoline than our great grandparents got during their entire lifetime. The toxicity problem is worldwide and includes heavy metals, radiation and industrial waste. Food is also a big source. The average person takes in about 14 pounds of chemicals per year in the United States in the form of food additives, humectants, preservatives, and food colorings. These toxins have to be cleared out of the body, if the body is going to restore its health, and there are various cleansing methods that work very well.

Energy Field Imbalances Is The Fifth Type Of Imbalance.

The energy field that is within us is highly organized into:

1. Circuits which are like the fuses in a house,

2. Systems which are groups of circuits and

3. Chakras which are deep energy centers.

These circuits and systems and chakras can become imbalanced or short-circuited. If they become imbalanced, then they need to be fixed if the body is going to recover.

What we are really talking about here is the energetic body that is within us. Anciently, this was called the prana or the chi. It is the template that our physical body fills into. This part of us may become imbalanced. Our physical body fills into the energetic template that this internal energy field provides. Organs and glands which become imbalanced internally in the body can be detected by touching points that we call BodyCode points, or test points on the surface of the body and through muscle testing, it can be determined if these organs or glands are balanced or imbalanced energetically.

Here is a representation of some of the BodyCode test points.

Each point corresponds to an organ or gland. By touching a point and performing a muscle test, we can test the balance of the organs and glands. If we touch the gallbladder point, for example, and the arm weakness on testing, it indicates an electrical or energetic imbalance in the gallbladder. In other words, at some point the gallbladder has 'blown its fuse' or has 'short-circuited.' When that happens, a muscle in the right knee will also become imbalanced. That will tend to lead to joint imbalance in the right knee, and the result will probably be pain in the right knee at some point in the future.

Correcting the gallbladder imbalance will immediately also correct the muscle imbalance in the knee. This is one of the ways that the body can be helped to return to normal function. By restoring balance to the organs, we restore balance to the muscles.

If the liver becomes overloaded for some reason, it may 'short-circuit' or 'blow its fuse.' If that happens, a certain muscle in the middle of the back called the rhomboid muscle will immediately imbalance. This will cause instability in the joints between the shoulder blades and will tend to cause pain in the upper back in that area. When the liver is imbalanced, we also will tend to see allergies as the liver makes up the bulk of the immune system.

Just above the appendix, there is a valve in the colon known as the ileocecal valve. If this valve becomes short circuited, it will affect muscles deep in the pelvis on the right side. This will lead to low back pain, possibly also right hip pain, and even false allergies. False allergies occur when the ileocecal valve is imbalanced and the body no longer is eliminating poisons as well as it should. As a result, toxins back up into the blood stream and a sinus drainage condition is created. When we correct the ileocecal valve, the sinus drainage often immediately goes away.

Kidney imbalances often lead to pain in the low back, in the hips, and even in the neck as well as fatigue. In Chinese medicine, the kidneys are energy reservoirs and they can become imbalanced due to drinking too much coffee or to a variety of other toxins. This will tend to cause imbalance in the muscles that support the lower lumbar spine as well as muscles that support the neck. In 17 years of practice, I never saw a single disc injury patient without an accompanying kidney imbalance. In all that time, I only had to send out two patients for surgical intervention, because if we correct the kidney imbalance, we thereby correct the muscle imbalance, which corrects the spinal imbalance, and the back can return into its normal state.

So now we have covered infections/infestations, structural misalignment, nutritional imbalances, toxicity, and energy field imbalances.

Many of the more chronically ill patients that I saw were suffering from imbalance in all of these areas. In other words, every piece of the puzzle that you see here is imbalanced in some people. Some people just have one or two of these areas imbalanced, **but** the bottom line is that if you are going to get well, what you have to do is find out what imbalances you have, and you have to fix those imbalances.

There is only one way that this can be done. The Unihipili (subconscious mind) must be accessed in order to determine what the body really needs. This is done through muscle testing, or another method of testing as described earlier.

Trapped Emotions Is The Sixth Type Of Imbalance.

Glenn's note: Whether you choose a method to heal, transmute and release *feelings* and emotions based on Bradley Nelson, John Ruskan or someone else, heal, transmute and release *both trapped and suppressed or repressed feelings* and emotions. Also, as you heal you will become able to clear *feelings* and emotions when it is best to wait. Bradley Nelson asks "Do I have a trapped emotion I can release now?". I suggest you ask, "Do I have a trapped or suppressed *feeling* or emotion it is best I heal and release now?".

What are Trapped Emotions? They are distortions in the energy field caused by negative emotional energy that has become 'trapped' in the body. These can be found and released magnetically by using a process I call "The Emotion Code," which is explained fully in my book by the same name.

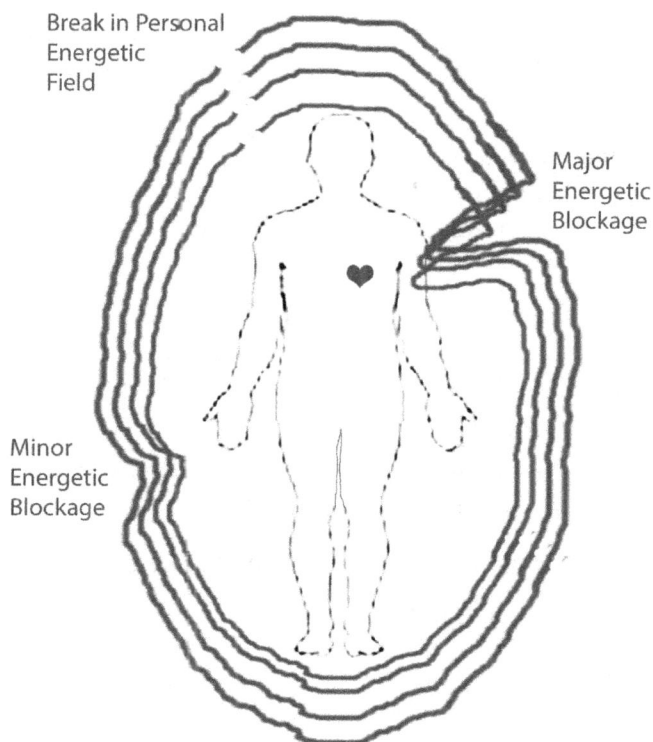

Think of the picture above as an egg shaped oblate spheroid (egg-shaped sphere) completely surrounding you.

Notice in the picture how this person's magnetic field (represented by the blue lines) is being distorted by trapped emotions. Notice the break in the field. If the trapped emotion and block is severe enough a hole can actually be torn in the field. In reality, trapped emotions are invisible to the naked eye, and consist of pure emotional energy.

Trapped emotions can occur at any age, and they can even be inherited.

A trapped emotion is an imbalance that will cause inflammation in the tissues, congestion, and more. These can be found and released quite easily from the body using "The Emotion Code."

It is difficult for me to express to you how wide spread and what a major problem trapped emotions are in our society. They cause phobias and I have seen many phobias corrected instantly using the Emotion Code. I have seen thousands of cases where acute physical pain instantly disappeared with the release of a Trapped Emotion. I have seen patients who were extremely depressed who completely recovered within just a matter of days.

Animals also suffer from Trapped Emotions, and I have many stories where animals have been helped quite dramatically by releasing their emotions as well.

HeartWall

One of the biggest breakthroughs that I have ever made is regarding what I have come to call the HeartWall™. Sometimes, trapped emotions can cluster around the heart. The heart is the core of your being.

New research reveals that the heart is actually a second brain that has memory and thinks. When you fall in love, you use your heart-brain. When someone really hurts you, you may *feel* like you have been hit in the chest; this sensation is where words like 'heartache' and 'heartbreak' actually come from.

Sometimes, emotions trapped in this area will form into a 'Heart-Wall' which blocks your love from getting out to other people, as well as blocking others' love from getting in to you. A Heart-Wall will prevent you from being able to live a full and complete life.

When we find the *feelings* and emotions that make up the Heart-Wall and heal, transmute and release the negative, and integrate the positive counterpart, amazing things happen. Wonderful things happen when we heal and dissolve the heart wall.

Sometimes trapped emotions can become lodged around the heart, and can create a 'Heart-Wall.'

Have you ever been injured emotionally? Have you ever *felt* that emotional heaviness in your chest like your heart was breaking?

The heart is the center of your being. In fact, research now indicates that the heart may be a second brain, a brain more powerful than the one on top of your shoulders. A brain that is fully activated when you are giving and receiving pure love and acts of pure, unselfish devotion. It is through our heart that we give and receive love.

But our hearts are vulnerable to emotional injury. Sometimes trapped emotions are created in the body, and sometimes these trapped emotions lodge in the heart area.

Since all things are nothing **but** pure energy by their very nature, a trapped emotion is no different, and consists of pure energy.

Well, sometimes your Unihipili (subconscious mind) will take that extra energy that is now in the heart area, and it will literally make a 'wall' with it. Why? To protect your heart from injury; to keep your heart from being totally broken.

I believe that Heart Walls affect us in two ways. First, they block the heart energy from flowing through the body; this makes it more difficult for the body to heal itself, and can cause physical symptoms, particularly in the neck, upper back and shoulders. Second, they block us from fully opening our hearts to others.

In essence, a HeartWall will make you numb to others and make it more difficult for you to *feel* emotions and connect to others. When you realize that the mind puts the heart wall up to protect us in the first place, it all makes sense, **but** if you have a HeartWall, you will have a harder time being able to give and receive love freely.

When the Heart Wall is removed from the body, the difference can sometimes be *felt* immediately. At other times, the change is more subtle and takes place over time. One of the main reasons that I teach my BodyCode Seminars, and the main reason I wrote "The Emotion Code" is the Heart-Wall phenomenon. I can never hope to clear enough HeartWalls in my lifetime to make a very big difference to the world. **But** if enough individuals learn how to heal, transmute and release these emotions, many hearts can be "unlocked", and the level of love and understanding in the world will increase. In this small way, maybe we really can change the world.

Adapted by author from Dr. Bradley Nelson's web site around 2009 when this information was downloadable for free. The web page is no longer available as of February 14, 2014. His current web site is <http://www.drbradleynelson.com/>.

Magnetism And Using Magnets To Heal And Release Trapped Feelings And Emotions

Bio-North And South Poles — The True Difference

Magnetic research has revealed that the bio-north and south pole energies from a magnet have an opposite effect on your body and its cells. Doctors recommend that pain, inflammation, bruising, infection, and most other applications require the use of the bio-north pole. The south pole could stimulate bacteria, viruses and cancer, therefore the south pole is avoided.

Because each cell in your body carry electrical charges, the bio-north polarity magnets will influence the electrical charge of your cells to a negative (north pole) ionic charge. This is the state that your cells are in when they are properly oxygenated, pH balanced and healthy. A positively charged cell creates and requires low oxygen, over acidity and swelling or edema

Quoting Dr. Richard Broeringmeyer:

"It has been clinically established that north pole energy arrests protein activity, draws fluids, contracts, vaso-constricts, increases alkalinity, acts to sedate or inhibit pain, decreases activity, increases potassium ions, decreases abnormal calcium ions and decreases hydrogen ion concentration. The north pole can be said to be the normalizing energy. It normalizes the alkaline state of the body **but** never produces an over alkalinized condition. It oxygenates the body **but** never produces oxidized free radicals. It has a normalizing effect no matter how long the exposure."

Behind The Science of Magnetics

Humans are dependent on an external source of magnetism. This was proven in the 1960's when astronauts required the use of magnets to replace the magnetic field of the Earth. Before the use of supplemental magnetism, space travelers experienced up to 80% loss of bone calcium. Proper magnetic therapy has been proven to enhance the body's natural ability to be healthy and heal itself, instead of just masking symptoms as many other treatments do in our modern day world. On its own, the body treats injury and illness with magnetic energy, which it derives from within itself (Krebs Cycle) and from the Earth's magnetic field.

It has been established that the magnetic field of the Earth, on which our bodies depend, has been decreasing. It has decreased from a level of over 4 gauss, 4,000 years ago, to less than 1/2 gauss today(5). People are currently healthier in parts of the earth where magnetic fields are stronger. George J. Washnis (2) reports that millions of people annually visit Lourdes, France, where greater magnetic fields prevail. As a result of bathing, drinking, and dabbing the water of

Lourdes on their body, "All seem to *feel* better as pain and stress are relieved, while over 2,000 inexplicable cures (with 65 so-called miracles) have been recognized by the authorities."

As part of the circle of optimum health you should sleep on a Lyon Legacy Gold or Silver Series Magnetic Mattress Pad. This pad can help to heal, restore, and revitalize your body while you sleep, when your body is in its natural state of healing and restoration. For specific health concerns apply a properly designed Lyon Legacy therapeutic magnetic product to the affected area of your body.

Clinical observations of Dr. William Philpott and others

North Pole - Negative Polarity (-)	South Pole - Positive Polarity (+)
fights infection	accelerates microorganism growth
relieves pain	increases pain
reduces inflammation	can increase inflammation
encourages restorative sleep	stimulates wakefulness
increases cellular oxygen	decreases cellular oxygen
normalizes acid balance	encourages high acid levels
supports biological healing	inhibits biological healing
reduces fluid retention	increases edema
pulls fluids and gases	pushes fluids and gases
reduces fatty deposits	encourages fatty deposits

How Magnets Can Help

To BETTER UNDERSTAND how magnetics can help relieve pain it is helpful to understand some of the causes of pain and illness.

Magnetic therapy enhances your body's utilization of healthful foods and herbal supplements, and makes exercise and physical therapy more effective.

Because each cell in your body carries electrical charges, the bio-north polarity magnets will influence the electrical charge of your cells to a negative (north pole) ionic charge. This is the state that your cells are in when they are properly oxygenated, pH balanced and healthy. Since this state of health may be a change from what is normal for you, occasionally, pain may increase at first. This is normally a sure sign that the magnetism is working in the body. If pain increases, simply remove the magnet if needed, allow the body to stabilize, then reapply the magnet or try it in a different location near the area originally treated. We recommend that you continue proper bio-north magnetic therapy for a period of time even if you see no instant results. or if symptoms or pain are increased initially. Remember that bio-north pole magnetism is completely safe and the goal is much more than temporary pain relief. If unsure as to how to proceed with questions specifically related to your health, contact your doctor.

Sleeping on one of our properly-designed bio-north polarity mattress pads creates a 4-6 gauss magnetic field from the magnets. Four gauss is what has been established as the level that the earth was at when the energy was ideal for health and healing. Sleeping on this 4-6 gauss field can safely restore and "Super Charge" your body and its cells each night through encouraging better sleep, oxygenating your body and encouraging a proper alkalized pH balance.

One in three Americans use alternative therapies and hundreds of thousands use magnetic therapy. Worldwide, over 100 million people use this therapy, 30 million in Japan alone, where 10 million people sleep on magnetic beds to counter the effects of stress, pain, fatigue and various ailments.

The Food and Drug Administration approved the use of electromagnets for medical purposes in 1978 and considers the permanent magnet even safer. Over 100,000 operations for bone fusion, muscular disorders, and other serious ailments are performed with electromagnets by licensed orthopedic surgeons annually. Permanent magnets do essentially the same work as electromagnets, without the side effects and expense that are associated with this alternating magnetism.

Infections And Magnets:

Infections are acidic and can be quickly neutralized by bio-north magnetism. This treatment normalizes pH, corrects cellular swelling (edema), promotes oxygenation, and actually has an antibiotic effect on microorganisms. It is important to remember that in treating an infection, often the bio-north magnet will relieve the symptoms in as quickly as a few minutes. It is recommended, however, to continue the treatment for a minimum of 14 days to achieve the full antibiotic effect. Magnetized water is an excellent, very effective way to treat an infection both externally and internally (orally) on an ongoing basis.

Adapted by author from <https://www.lyonlegacy.com/learn/north_south.aspx> (12/21/2013)

Which Magnet To Use:

North Pole Curved Magnet by Lyon Legacy International as used by person who introduced me to the 'The Emotion Code'.

This is the magnet I use.

Flexible - 2 1/4 x 3 1/2 - Item #: 608

<https://www.lyonlegacy.com/wexec/order.exe/item?no=845>

Takes you to item #608)12/21/2013)

1 (888) 205-3422   Retail Price: $11.95

or

Nikken as recommended by Bradley Nelson

Biaxial PowerMag - $250 as of 1/10/2014

<http://nettrax.myvoffice.com/nikkenusa/ShoppingCart/Shop.cfm?
CurrPage=CategoryDetail&NextPage=CategoryDetail&CategoryID=422&lng=eng&shiptocount
ry=USA&pwp=>

MagCreato - $190 as of 1/10/2014

<http://nettrax.myvoffice.com/nikkenusa/ShoppingCart/Shop.cfm?
CurrPage=CategoryDetail&NextPage=CategoryDetail&CategoryID=55&lng=eng&shiptocountr
y=USA&pwp=>

Kenko MagDuo - $78 as of 1/10/2014

<http://nettrax.myvoffice.com/nikkenusa/ShoppingCart/Shop.cfm?
CurrPage=CategoryDetail&NextPage=CategoryDetail&CategoryID=650&lng=eng&shiptocount
ry=USA&pwp=>

As you become attuned to Source a magnet becomes unnecessary. You can use the energy of LOVE coming through your hands.

Using The Emotion Code

If you have no trapped or inherited trapped emotions that it is best to clear now, there are several possibilities.

The **first possibility** is that the subject has no trapped emotions at all. This is very unlikely, since nearly everyone has them.

The **second possibility** may be that the subject has a trapped emotion, **but** for some reason their *Unihipili (*subconscious mind*)* is resistant to releasing it right now. This was the statement: "I have a trapped emotion that it is best I release now". The subject may be willing, **but** their Unihipili (SubConscious mind) may need time. Divine Wisdom and the Unihipili may know it is better to wait. This situation can change, and the answer may be different later on.

The **third possibility** is that the subject has a Heart-Wall. If this is the case, the body may say that there are no trapped emotions, when in reality there are. The Heart-Wall has the effect of making all trapped emotions a little harder to find.

A Heart-Wall is made by the Unihipili (subconscious mind) to protect your heart; it must protect your delicate core in any way it can. The Heart-Wall may have many layers.

You heal/dissolve the Heart-Wall by healing, transmuting and releasing the trapped emotions that created the Heart-Wall.

If you are struggling with a specific problem in your life, it's important to determine if trapped emotions may be playing an unseen role. You might suspect that you have a trapped emotion and yet when you ask the general question, "Do I have a trapped emotion that it is best I heal and release now?", you get an answer of *no*. Trapped emotions sometimes need to be addressed more directly for them to unveil themselves.

Adapted by author from Dr. Bradley Nelson's web site around 2009 when this was downloadable for free. The web page is no longer available as of February 14, 2014. His current web site is <http://www.drbradleynelson.com/>.

'Soul Echoes' and "The Emotion Code"

Adapted by author from Dr. Bradley Nelson's web site around 2009 when this was downloadable for free. The web page is no longer available as of February 14, 2014. His current web site is <http://www.drbradleynelson.com/>.

Glenn's thoughts are on this and the next page. The Actual Exercise is after the explanation.

You may have very subtle or strong visuals and emotional responses. Just do the exercise with Love, have faith, and allow the Divine Flow. Healing has taken place, even if the conscious mind is unaware of it. Conscious awareness will come.

What causes one part of the body to be healthy and another part to be diseased? What causes emotional and mental instability? It can be a chemical or nutritional imbalance or a physical injury. It can also be energetic.

The distortions, mutations and all lower vibration (dense) disharmonic thought forms from what we perceive as past moments can be thought of as *miasms*, *'cellular memory'*, *'Imprints On The Luminous Energy Field'*, *memories replaying, beliefs, soul contracts, and agreements* that are no longer in harmony with our highest good. All of these, and more, can be thought of as *'**Soul Echoes**'* to be released. There is no need to forget them. Keep the information and release the patterns.

'**Soul Echoes**' are concepts, decisions, attitudes, alignments, truths, contracts, oaths, agreements, vows and unresolved emotions held in your conscious and unconscious fields or awareness that we are living by and have made with other people or ourselves. Some are over thousands of years old. These '**Soul Echoes**' create and magnetize lower frequency events and experiences in our current incarnate reality and cause the mutations in our physical DNA as well as emotional and mental challenges. Physical toxins and impurities from our environment and diet can also cause disease and damage to the DNA.

Our current life situations are not only created through our past and present choices. We inherit imprints from our past lives, parents and ancestors at conception. We also inherit them from Mother Earth and the collective. Since we have simultaneous incarnations in different time/space zones which are all connected to one template, we also have karmic bleed through from our eleven soul extensions (parallel selves) who are still in incarnation. This bleed through can emerge from the past or future. An example of this is that karmic bleed through can manifest as physical symptoms being experienced that are not in truth your own. If another soul extension (parallel self) is experiencing something, you can be experiencing this same 'thing' through your physical body.

When we clear the 'Soul Echoes' we clear the time line and destiny of all our selves.

Allow the highest priority '**Soul Echoes**' to clear as Spirit chooses. You may think of a specific challenge/symptom you want to work on. If you do, let go of expectations and the thinking and allow Spirit to do the clearing and healing.

The clearing of blockages progressively purges ancient distortions and mutations.

Once this negative 'data' is removed any resulting voids need to be filled.

Remember:

As you heal you will become able to clear 'Soul Echoes', *feelings* and emotions when it is best to wait.

Bradley Nelson asks "Do I have a trapped emotion *I can* release now?"

I suggest you ask, "Do I have a 'Soul Echo' **it is best** I heal and release now?"

In some way the 'Soul Echoes' are held in place by emotions and *feelings* and the emotions and *feelings* are energized by the 'soul echoes'. This exercise is one way to heal, clear and release both.

Note: Bradley Nelson uses a bio-north magnet to heal and clear the distortion and facilitate the clearing. You can use a magnet or your own way of clearing when you get to step 5.

When I use a magnet I use a magnet from <https://www.lyonlegacy.com/wexec/order.exe/item?no=845> Flexible - 2 1/4 x 3 1/2 - Item #: 608. Takes you to item #608)12/21/2013). Retail Price: $11.95. It is inexpensive and effective.

The "Emotion Code' Actual Exercise begins here

The following Flow Chart created by author is based on *The Emotion Code* by Bradley Nelson

	Ask Permission First		
	Question	Answer/Action	Answer/Action
1	Ask: Do You (I) have a *'Soul Echo'* it is best We (I) Release now?	If YES go to 2	If NO go to 1-a
1-a	Ask: Is it best We (I) release a *'Soul Echo'* from a Heart-Wall now?	If YES go to 2	If NO go to 1-b
1-b	Ask: Is it best We (I) release a *'Soul Echo'* from a Hidden Heart-Wall now?	If YES go to 2	If NO go to 1-c
1-c	Ask: Is it best We (I) release a *'Soul Echo'* from before conception now?	If YES go to2	If NO go to 1-d
1-d	Is it best We (I) release a *'Soul Echo'* about a specific person, event, situation, action, thought, belief, memory or problem now?	If YES Investigate & then go to 2	If NO go to 2
2	Determine Correct Column on Next Page	Colum A or Colum B	
	Determine Correct Row on Next Page	Row 1, 2, 3, 4, 5 or 6	
	Determine exact *'Soul Echo'* emotion on Next Page (5 Emotions per cell) (example A:3:3 would be Column A, Row 3, 3rd emotion in the cell	Then go to 3	
3	Is it best if I know more?	If YES go to 4	If NO go to 5
4	Is it my *'Soul Echo'*? Is it inherited? Did I take on someone's *'Soul Echo'*? Is it best I know when it became lodged? Is it best I know where the trapped *'Soul Echo'* is lodged?	If any of these are YES investigate and then go to 4-a	If NO go to 4-a
4-a	Is it best if I know more?	If YES go to 4-b	If NO go to 5
4-b	Keep investigating – When there is no need to know more go to 5		
5	Move **bio-north** magnet with north pole towards the body from 1st Chakra, up torso, over head and down to base of skull **3x** (**10 x for inherited).**	Then go to 6	
6	Did we heal and release the *'Soul Echo'*?	If YES: go to 7	If NO: Re-Check
7	**"Is it best if we (I) heal and release another *Soul Echo* at this time.?"**	If YES: Go back to 1	If NO: Done for now

Awareness - A Path to Spiritual and Physical Health and Well-Being

Chart Of Emotions To Use With 'The Emotion Code'

The chart below is from Dr. Bradley Nelson's web site around 2009 when this was downloadable for free. The web page is no longer available as of February 14, 2014. His current web site is <http://www.drbradleynelson.com/>.

	Organ or System Affected	Feelings/Emotions generated by 'Soul Echoes' and holding 'Soul Echoes' in place	
		Column A feeling/emotion	Column B feeling/emotion
Row 1	Heart or Small Intestine	Rejection /Abandonment	Effort Unreceived / Need for Approval
		Betrayal	Heartache
		Forlorn	Insecurity
		Lost	Overjoy
		Love Unreceived	Vulnerability
Row 2	Spleen or Stomach	Anxiety	Failure
		Despair	Helplessness
		Disgust	Hopelessness
		Nervousness	Lack of Control
		Worry	Low Self-Esteem
Row 3	Lung or Colon	Crying	Confusion
		Discouragement	Defensiveness
		Rejection	Grief
		Sadness	Self-Abuse
		Sorrow	Stubbornness
Row 4	Liver or Gall Bladder	Anger/Rage	Depression
		Bitterness	Frustration
		Guilt	Indecisiveness
		Hatred	Panic
		Resentment	Taken for Granted
Row 5	Kidneys or Bladder	Blaming	Conflict
		Dread	Creative Insecurity
		Fear	Terror
		Horror	Unsupported
		Peeved	Wishy Washy/Uncertainty
Row 6	Glands and Sexual Organs	Humiliation	Pride
		Jealousy	Shame/Need to be Judged
		Longing	Shock
		Lust	Unworthy
		Overwhelmed	Worthless

Healing, Transmuting, Releasing And Integrating Suppressed *Feelings* And Emotions

This section is based on *The Emotional Clearing Process* by John Ruskan and elaborated in his 2003 book, *Emotional Clearing: An East/West Guide to Releasing Negative Feelings and Awakening Unconditional Happiness*.

Introduction To The Emotional Clearing Process

"Are you ready for real inner healing?"

Are you trying to sort out all the possible options of the New Age, and starting to see that the ultimate happiness you seek is unattainable by simplistic positive thinking or by just visualizing what you want?

Do you hunger for psychologically substantial in-depth information and super-effective guidance as you contend with vital personal issues concerning your well-being and life's purpose?

Are you unsure of how to proceed or are you overwhelmed as you approach working with Eckhart Tolle's Pain Body?

Are you considering psychotherapy, or have you been involved with intellectual therapies that were ineffective or ignored the emotional level, leaving you with undeveloped emotional skills and unresolved *feelings*?

Have you been on the spiritual path, inadvertently bypassing negative emotions, **but** now realize that you must heal on the emotional level in order to continue consciousness growth, and your spiritual discipline is unable to offer meaningful guidance without dealing with negative *feelings*?

What The Emotional Clearing Process Will Do For You

Based on a unique fusion of proven Eastern spiritual and Western psychological principles, ECP provides you with a powerful, easy-to-use inner process that will enable you to heal, transmute and release the built-up, negative subconscious and integrate the positive.

You apply this process either on your own, or with assistance in the form of pre-recorded guided sessions, or with a live Emotional Clearing Facilitator.

The Emotional Clearing Process (ECP):

> An EAST/WEST inner-directed method for releasing negative *feelings* and awakening unconditional happiness.
> Teaches you how to heal, release and prevent negative *feelings* like fear, anger, hatred, jealousy, inadequacy, sexual issues, or depression from contaminating your life and relationships.
> Shows you how to manage your life so no more negative *feelings* are created by you to become trapped in the subconscious, building up and creating the PAIN BODY.
> Gives you a highly effective consciousness-based EAST/WEST self-therapy system that heals, transmutes and releases deep, trapped, Karmic negative *feelings*.
> Enables you to heal your emotional self as part of your spiritual practice.
> Empowers you to achieve goals by healing, transmuting and releasing inner blocking.
> Teaches you how to dissolve stress and learn to relax.

I know you want to find a way to improve yourself and your life. You want to make the most out of this short time we have on the earth. You want to evolve. You want to be happy. You want to go beyond struggle.

Many times, we think we need to attain some outer goal before we can be happy. We think that if we only had that perfect relationship with our spouse, lover, co-workers, or children, we'd be happy. Or if we only had that better job, more money, more recognition, more sex, and so on.

The real secret is that none of these things are needed to be happy. You just need to heal and release the negative *feelings* inside that you think the external things will make better.

You can heal these *feelings* directly to achieve lasting relief and UNCONDITIONAL HAPPINESS.

'Unconditional' means that your happiness comes from the inside, independent of the external.

The amazing thing is that as you start to heal and release negative *feelings* by going inside, you also start to release the BLOCKING that has been preventing you from achieving outer goals!

You find yourself more easily achieving outer goals, as if they are just being brought to you, and at the same time you become less compulsive about attaining the outer goals.

You become a well-balanced, non-compulsive, happy human being

ECP offers distinctive and well-informed insights about transformational psychology. For example, lately there's been a lot of talk about the Law of Attraction.

The Truth About The 'Law Of Attraction'

It's true that what you hold within creates your external experience, including what you attract to yourself. **But** this spiritual principle has been simplified and distorted in order to give it mass commercial appeal. Lately it's been taught that just by visualizing an image in your mind, or thinking the correct thoughts, you will attract what you want.

The way it really works is that it's the energy that's buried deep in the subconscious that attracts things to you. And if this energy is negative - painful, angry, fearful, full of failure, etc - that's what you draw to yourself.

The subconscious, as you've probably heard, is much vaster than the conscious mind, and therefore easily overpowers it. Simply holding positive thoughts in the conscious mind is unable to subdue the subconscious, and in fact, when you try to hold a positive image or thought in your mind which is contradicted by the subconscious, the subconscious negativity is stirred up and starts to work against you, attracting exactly the opposite of what you want!

The negative energy that is stored in the subconscious becomes known to us as *feelings* and emotions. That's why we emphasize healing, transmuting and releasing *feelings* and emotions as the means to releasing inner negativity.

Let Me Say It Again, Differently

When negative *feelings* are handled improperly, they get stored in latent form in what has come to be called "the subconscious," instead of healed and released. In Eckhart Tolle's terminology, this is the Pain Body. Even *feelings* from years, or life-times ago, are stored in the subconscious. Thoughts are missing this characteristic. And what exactly is stored?

Feelings are composed of energy, and as this energy continues to build in the subconscious, it starts to act out. It's the energy of the *feelings* that influences us, coloring our thoughts, beliefs, perceptions, our health, and eventually attracting negative circumstances.

Like attracts like; and it's the negative *feeling* energy in the subconscious that attracts negative circumstances. Negative *feelings* in the subconscious easily overpower any contrary thought that might be held in the conscious mind in order to attract positive conditions. We continue to attract negative conditions and experiences, based on the negative *feelings* trapped in the subconscious. In the East, this phenomenon is called Karma.

I have seen over and over, both in myself and the clients I work with, that favorable circumstances arise spontaneously when negative *feelings* are healed and released. There is no need to laboriously try to hold positive thoughts in the mind, which only adds to left-brain stress and a sense of becoming isolated in your mind, losing touch with reality, and increasing the ego-driven self-orientation which all true schools of consciousness development teach you to transcend.

In fact, because of the law of Duality, holding positive thoughts in the mind to try to counter negative *feeling* energies in the subconscious will only stir up those negative *feelings* and attract more negativity!

<u>The important thing to get is that trying to cultivate positive thoughts or *feelings* to replace or recondition the negative without releasing the negative is ineffective and often counterproductive. It can actually strengthen the negative.</u>

Negative *feelings* must be healed and released directly by some kind of process based on a sophisticated understanding of how the subconscious functions.

Adapted by author from <http://www.emclear.com/index.html>

Emotions And Addictions

This section is based on The Emotional Clearing Process by John Ruskan and elaborated in his 2003 book, *Emotional Clearing: An East/West Guide to Releasing Negative Feelings and Awakening Unconditional Happiness*.

The capacity for *feeling* and managing emotions is of utmost importance. Emotions are our connection to life; without them we are stale, hollow, and cut off from true fulfillment, **but** when they get out of control, we experience distress and discouragement.

Self-blocking occurs on the emotional level, rather than on the mental or intellectual level. The emotional level is where we are most unconscious. People who have achieved self-acceptance and emotional mastery have developed the capacity for *feeling* deeply, without resistance, whatever is happening in their inner life. Most of us, instead of doing this, block *feelings* from entering consciousness, resulting in emotional imbalance and confusion.

SubstanceAddiction/Abuse:

Substance addiction, whether to drugs, alcohol, smoking, or food, is a form of escape. The addictive cycle provides psychic energy that is used to maintain suppression as well as to provide energy to simply function. This condition is reached because of the habitual behavior of escaping. The constant turning away from ourselves builds the blocks that cut us off from our natural, inner energy resources, resulting in extreme self-rejection and dependence on the substance.

In all substance abuse, we gain access to energy within. What we tap into, however, is a form of reserve energy. We use up our reserves, and the eventual end is complete psychic and physical exhaustion. Addiction to alcohol as well as to illegal and prescription drugs is rampant in our culture, although many people think they have no addiction because their level of consumption is no more than normal. They see themselves as "social" drinkers or drug users. In other forms of addiction, we tap into energy outside of ourselves. This happens in power or sexual addictions, for example, when others are involved.

All addictions have the same deceptive quality. We think we are benefiting from the addiction because we *feel* more relaxed or function better when we are on the peak. We forget that the valleys between the peaks are also created by the addictive cycle.

Addiction:

A center is considered integrated when there is a balanced experience of the dualistic qualities of that center. This means we have learned to recognize and accept both the "positive" and "negative" poles of the duality, incorporating them into a basically positive experience. No large amount of avoidance and suppression is occurring, and previously suppressed energies have been healed and cleared. If we are unable to realistically say that we have learned to experience the negative pole in a harmonious way, at least we have learned how to accept it and use it constructively – for example, through processing.

We Become Addicted To The Positive Because We Are Unwilling To Face The Negative

Unintegrated, we become addicted at various levels of experience. We become addicted to the "positive" side of any one dualistic experience because we are unwilling to face the "negative" side of its duality. We seek to escape to the positive side, often unaware that both sides are dependent on one another for their existence.

However, because of the nature of dualism, the more we try to experience the positive, the more we also generate the negative. We become frustrated. We attempt to suppress the intensifying negative with more experiences of the positive, and the addiction cycle builds. Addiction can occur in all centers as well as at the Sensation or Nurturing levels, where it is normally recognized. We develop a deep hunger for a particular need, **but** no matter what we do to try to satisfy the hunger, it remains or even becomes worse. Addictive behavior is also known as "compulsive."

Addiction Requires Psychic Energy

Each addiction can be related to a certain center of consciousness. Addiction is the result of an energy imbalance in that particular center. The center is at least partially blocked and unlike in a healthy center, normal energy flow is blocked. The center is blocked because of our suppression. Through the avoidance of *feelings* in the center, we create the block. To maintain the block requires energy, energy the addiction supplies. All addiction provides an extra supply of energy, taken either from external sources or from the body's internal reserves.

The cravings that arise for a particular object of addiction are learned. Through experience, we learn that energy can be obtained from a certain source and used to maintain the block. When the block begins to weaken, because the suppressing energy is getting low, we begin to get glimpses of exactly what we are suppressing, and we experience discomfort, anxiety, depression, and so on. We then seek the addictive experience once more, to gain the energy required to maintain the block to the *feelings*. The *feelings* are re-suppressed, over and over. Because the suppressed *feelings* will continue to build, the suppressing energy also must keep increasing, resulting in the extraordinary means that must be used to provide the energy. We enter the expanding cycle of addiction.

Usually we are addicted to a center's complement to the negative experience. However, we also can escape to another, usually higher, center and draw energy from there. The higher center will suppress the pain of the lower center. Thus, if we experience anxiety from an unintegrated Survival center, we could attempt to suppress it by becoming compulsively addicted to wealth and security, **but** we also could suppress it by compulsive seeking in any higher center, such as sex, power, love, even creativity.

The first step in breaking addiction is to understand how it works. When you know why you act compulsively, you weaken the power of the addiction. You must stop yielding to the addictive experience. Process the addictive urge as well as the *feeling* that you are suppressing with the addiction. Self-processing can be the main approach, **but** other approaches, such as therapy, group support, or medical support in cases of chemical dependency, are helpful as well.

When you confront *feelings* related to addiction, you meet your demon head on. You must realize that you are healing and releasing accumulated negativity; proceed patiently and gently as well as sensibly. Avoid demanding too much of yourself and avoid yielding too easily. The delicate balance, the sense of making steady progress, must be established. As you learn how to heal yourself, you will acquire new tools that will help you tremendously. You will be able to cleanse negativity that previously compelled you to act in addictive ways.

Further Explanation Of Suppression of Emotions by John Ruskin

There are descending influences (trauma to a higher center/level causes problems in the lower centers/levels) and ascending influences (trauma to a lower center/level causes problems in the upper centers/levels). Therefore true healing requires simultaneous healing on all levels.

I believe the following process functions on all levels simultaneously. You need to take the appropriate action at the physical level, so this may require conscious choices/decisions to minimize/limit and eventually eliminate the physical influences that can cause problems in the upper centers/levels

Although there are many energy centers in the body, usually only seven are considered to be of major importance. However, in practice I have found it helpful to use a slightly more comprehensive schematic of the chakra system, giving a total of ten. The location of these additional centers was first suggested to me by the Taoist chakra system, **but** the psychological qualities I have assigned to them are based on my own observations..

Using the additional points clarifies the confusion and ambiguity that I previously found in dealing with qualities traditionally attributed to the Solar Plexus, Heart, and Throat chakras. The new points are the Power, Nurturing, and Creative centers. Each of the ten points corresponds to one of the ten planets, giving a revealing correlation between the chakras and the astrological birth chart, which can be a useful tool for healing.

The Chakras Are Where Our Blocks Are Located

(Glenn's note: I find it more inclusive to use the concept of "Centers of Consciousness. The concept of chakras seems limiting. See table and graphic below.)

When we suppress an unpleasant *feeling*, we interrupt the natural flow of energies instead of allowing the *feeling* to clear itself, to resolve itself, to regain its natural equilibrium. The energy becomes trapped, held in storage in a static condition. Where does the energy get stored? It is held in what has come to be called "the subconscious.

Remember ALL your choices affect everyone, all your chakras and 'ALL THAT IS'.

15 Chakras And Energy Centers - Table and graphic below created by author

Five Methods of Healing, Clearing and Releasing

# on Drawing	Location	Standard Chakra	John Ruskan	Kay C. Whitaker	Comment
1	Below the feet			Below the Feet	Moves a lot
2	Bottom of feet			Bottom of each foot	
3	Knees			Knees	
4	Base of spine	1-Root	1-Survival Center		
5	Between anus and vagina or testicles		2-Power Center		Controlling or giving power away
6	Hips			Hips	Smaller centers at hips move - sometimes outside the body
7	Below the Belly Button	2-Sacral	3- Sensation Center		Sensuality/Sexuality
8	Naval		4-Nurturing Center		
9	About one inch below the breast bone	3-Solar Plexus	5-Significance Center	Upper Belly	Smaller centers move. Psychological home of the ego
10	Center of Chest	4-Heart	6-Heart Center	Heart	
11	Throat, Mouth and Ears	5-Throat (Throat only)	7-Expression Center (Throat only)	Mouth, Ears and Throat	
12	Base of Skull in back		9-Creative Center		
13	Physical Eyes and Center of Forehead	6-Third Eye (center of forehead only)	8-Intuitive/Witness Center (center of forehead only)	Eyes	Can move a great deal. Sometimes expands itself into the center at the top of the head
14	Just outside the body, above the head	7-Crown	10-Spiritual Center	Just above the head	
15	Hands			Hands	Expand and shrink and move all around, even into other realms

I believe there are many more Chakras/Energy Centers than these fifteen; possibly an infinite number. These are the fifteen I work with. They are all affected by our choices.

Any more than these, I turn over to my Unihipili (subconscious), my super conscious and Spirit.

Use your own perception and awareness for any clarification and refinement.

The drawing below was created by the author

Notice that I used colors other than those normally associated with the seven most commonly known chakras. ALL chakras incorporate all colors. A specific color may be primary to a specific chakra.

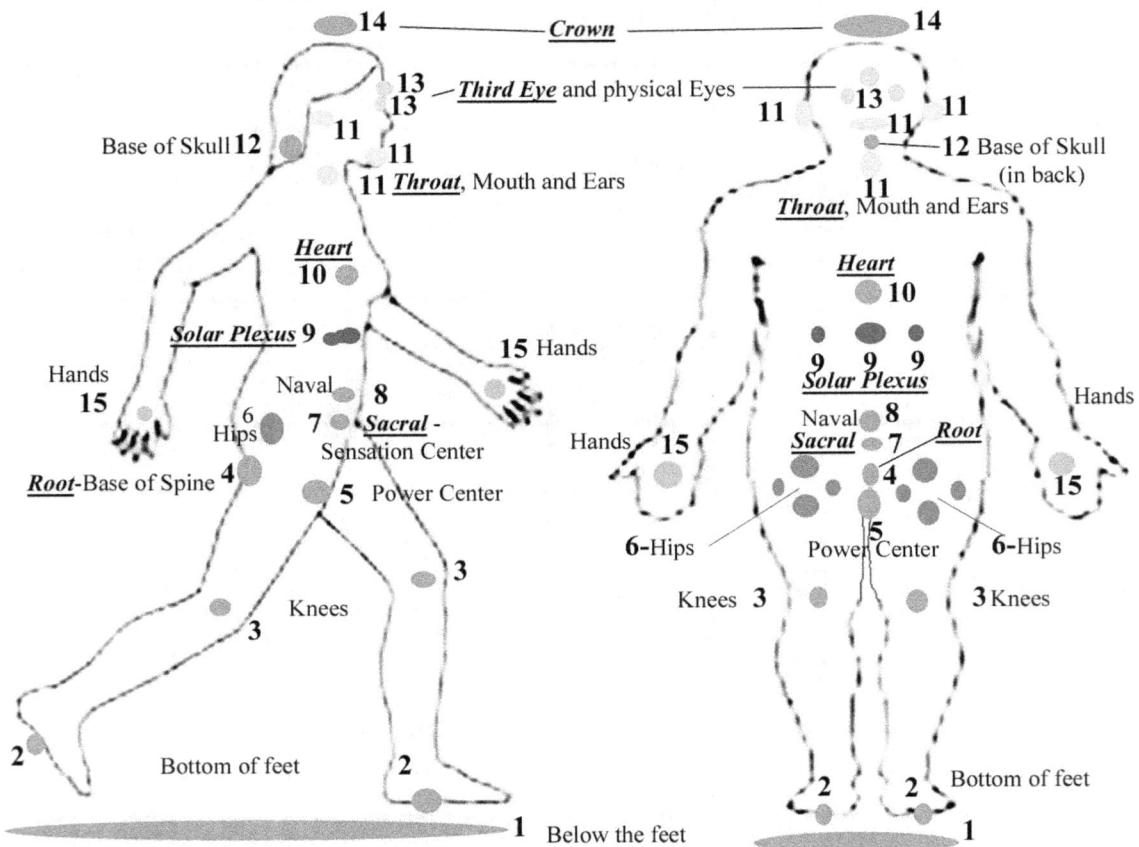

Suppression Creates Subconscious Karma

There is no way to heal, transmute and release traumatic *feelings* except by ending resistance to them and experiencing them, which was avoided when the event occurred. You must carefully watch how you reject and resist the *feelings*. Enter meditation, activate the Witness, and drop resistance; allow the *feelings* just to be. Let go of all blame. Allow them their own cycle and they will eventually dissolve as is best. Try to distinguish your thoughts from your *feelings*. Often there is a strong component of blame present in thoughts. This is all that is needed to prevent acceptance. You then remain unable to heal and release the *feelings* that are trapped in the energy body.

Allow Suppressed *Feelings* To Emerge

In meditation, brainwave frequency slows down to the alpha level of activity or lower, inducing relaxation and healing. If you heal, transmute, release and integrate in alpha, you have a tremendous advantage. Integration proceeds almost by itself, and the Witness is easily activated. Direct experience of *feelings* can be best accomplished in alpha during meditation (although it also can be done in activity, when the event is taking place). When you first sit to meditate, you may unaware of *feelings* that are affecting you because they are suppressed. When you allow yourself to enter the state of meditation as I described, suppressed *feelings* will spontaneously begin to jump into your awareness as the subconscious cleanses. Just sitting still gives the subconscious the opportunity to bring its suppressed contents to consciousness.

Two things happen when you sit quietly. The first is that your mind starts to go back into gear: doing, striving, planning, thinking, worrying. Usually no particularly intense *feeling* is associated with this kind of superficial activity. When you detect this superficial wandering of the mind, you are to gently stop such activity by reminding yourself that you are supposed to be doing nothing or by coming back to your focus point.

The second is that a suppressed *feeling* will come up. This occurrence is distinguished by the emergence of strong emotion. This is what you want. Recognize that healing and clearing is happening. Instead of turning from the *feeling* or going back to your focus point, stay with the *feeling* and with any associated thoughts or images, such as the interaction with another person. Move into a processing mode – own (welcome), accept, experience, witness, process and allow to heal, transmute, clear and integrate. Allow the *feeling* to remain in your consciousness until you *feel* a shift – until the *feeling* starts to link to another related *feeling* or diminishes.

Allow *Feelings* That Come Up In Meditation Instead Of Suppressing Them

When *feelings* come up in meditation, they must be handled properly if cleansing is to be effective. When I first began to meditate, I had no understanding of this. My intention in meditation was to calm the mind, expand my consciousness, and enter more blissful states – in other words, to escape.

Whenever disturbing emotions came up, I assumed I was having a bad meditation. I tried to avoid the *feelings* by bringing my attention back to my focus point. I became upset and would get angry about the anger, fearful about the fear, and so on. Meditation became a fight to try to control my thoughts and *feelings*. What I was doing, I understand now, was resuppressing negative energies that came up for healing and releasing. I had no concept of integration, as we have been discussing. I thought that eventually I would get past the negative intrusions. I never did, and I became pessimistic about meditation. I was unknowingly practicing what is called "suppressive meditation."

Eventually I came to understand that the problem was in my approach. This single insight had much to do with my decision to write this book, because I *feel* other people probably make the same mistake. By emphasizing integration and clearing, perhaps the pitfall of suppressive meditation can be avoided. When negative material comes up, in activity as well as in meditation, the subconscious is trying to heal and clear itself. You must take time to accept and experience whatever is surfacing. Even though I have been practicing meditation for most of my life, I have benefited most in recent years when I understood cleansing and allowed myself to be with negative *feelings*. Much, maybe most, of my meditation time is still spent healing, transmuting and clearing negative *feelings*.

When I sit to meditate now, I first enter alpha and the Witness. I go into my body. I start gentle breathing and watch for whatever body sensations may occur. I assume that any discomfort that appears in the body is just negative energies releasing themselves. I witness these. If I *feel* an emotion, I go into the corresponding center, breathing into the center to free the energy. I let the emotion or *feeling* build without reacting to it – I simply watch and *feel*. Soon that particular *feeling* will have dissipated and something else may come up. After a while, *feelings* and emotions will have spent themselves. I begin to lose awareness of the body and enter other stages of meditation. There is no fighting, no controlling, no intention, no expectation. I am fine with whatever happens.

Bring Up Past Unresolved Issues

Even though our main focus is on present *feelings* as they occur in response to our current life experiences, sometimes it is helpful to investigate and heal *feelings* about past events. Many painful, unresolved issues have a past-time reference. We have sustained hurt and loss in the past, and these *feelings* must be healed and released. Actually, we are still dealing with present *feelings*, and since they have a connection to the past, the *feelings* can be precipitated by going into the past. This is simply a therapeutic technique and is different than living in the past.

You can go back to any painful incident, recent or remote, and bring it into your field of awareness as you sit in meditation. See it before you. Allow the story to be told. Relive the incident from the Witness vantage point. Bring persons before you, in your meditation, who are important. Visualize emotionally charged scenes in your mind. The trapped subconscious pain will be triggered. As *feelings* come up, welcome them. If there are certain issues that you consider too painful to go into, they are obviously the very ones that need attention. They are likely to be influencing you in ways that are unsuspected. Other important areas of the past will become apparent to you. You will spontaneously see how past incidents connect with current problems.

Remember that you are trying to understand and learn from the past without going back into it. You are bringing up *feelings* for acceptance, experience, and integration. Allow understanding to come as a *result* of integration. Searching for understanding during meditation will prevent you from going into meditation, alpha, and the Witness. Remember to stay aware of the distinction between the *feeling* and the self-rejection that originally suppressed it. Deliberately drop the self-rejection. Be careful to avoid sitting and resuppressing the *feeling* by reliving the self-rejection.

Does It Matter If Memories Are "True"?

You may question whether going back into the past is pertinent to living your life now. It is, because the past becomes *symbolic* of the present. In a sense, it is unimportant if your memory is accurate or symbolic, and it will usually be symbolic; you are recalling your own subjective view, which may be very different from someone else's. Such recall is still effective because your memory is a symbolic drama, a metaphor, that triggers the subconscious.

You are doing therapy to yourself with this technique. Be unafraid of going deep into traumatic issues. Past events are the most common format in which *feelings* come up during meditation. Allow memories that recur without resisting them – it means that something is crying out for healing and release. Accept the memory, no matter how painful, and stay with it until all negativity is cleared. You can assume this has happened when there is no longer an emotional charge associated with the memory. If something is especially hard to face, it is a major issue for you and represents much more than you probably realize. Healing, transmuting and releasing it, will integrate more than you expect.

Accept Blocking

Sometimes, when we are trying to move into direct experience of a *feeling*, we get stuck and it seems that we can go no further. When this happens, usually we are coming face to face with our inner blocks themselves. Blocking occurs unconsciously; therefore it is difficult to undo it deliberately. At this point, we must move to *acceptance* of the blocking.

We allow ourselves to remain where we are as we sit in meditation – stuck. We accept being stuck. We watch it. We witness it. We process it. We accept where we are in our process instead of wishing we were somewhere else or further along.

Acceptance of the blocking is crucial to its releasing. Striving to overcome it only strengthens it, exactly like any other obstacle that we meet. When we accept, we lay the ground for the eventual loosening of the blocking. As we get to know the blocking more intimately, by allowing it to come more and more into consciousness, eventually it will open, without our asking, and we will move to direct experience of the *feelings* that have been hidden.

Bring Your *Feelings* To Crisis

If you enter the experience of a negative emotion and in any other way try to avoid the *feeling*, it may build within you. You may begin to tremble, *feeling* the energy as it moves around your body. You may become lost in emotion; your sense of identity may alter; you may begin weeping. By accepting a *feeling* or emotion instead of avoiding it you permit it to build to the point of crisis. This is the *healing crisis*. Instead of pursuing a *crisis* allow it. If it happens, you should know what to do.

Allowing your *feelings* to come to a crisis allows them to be 'let out' and released. Of course, *feelings* must be released instead of being allowed to accumulate in the energy body. Often, however, whatever method we choose for letting *feelings* out involves self-rejection. The *feelings* are then re-suppressed instead of being healed, let out and released.

When *feelings* are accepted, there is no suppression of them. The very act of keeping them in consciousness means they are being healed and cleared. If they can be kept in consciousness to the extent that a crisis builds, a catharsis and healing will follow. Allowing a crisis to build calls for the warrior spirit. Try it if the opportunity arises. You will push back some of your personal boundaries, I can assure you.

Emotional Clearing Process and How It Works

It's 1988. I'm at a point in my life of reassessment - of looking at where I am and wondering why I'm there. I've been earnestly "on the path" since the late sixties, so an important part of my self-evaluation concerns what we loosely call the "spiritual." Have I really achieved anything in the way of growth in the past 20 years? Am I succeeding in my efforts of self-realization? As I look honestly at myself, I see areas that call out in distress.

I see that I am often angry. I see that I experience much pain in intimate relationships. I see that I am isolated, lonely, and living in anxiety, and maybe, downright fear. All this even though I'm trying my best to keep up a dedicated meditation and Yoga practice, trying to be conscious of the Karma I am generating, trying to be a "loving and spiritual" person. One of the few consoling realizations is that I certainly have company. As I look at others, I see the same condition.

What I see is that we are all in emotional turmoil, including, and possibly especially, those of us on the consciousness path, because we are in the process of leaving behind old rigid structures that have served to keep us propped up and *feelings* held down and suppressed. It seems to me that if we could resolve these *feelings*, we would be doing something very important.

With regard to my personal path, I now see that resolving *feelings* is primary. I was taught to aim for higher consciousness, to become a loving and blissful person, **but** I was never taught how to handle the negative *feelings* inside as part of my spiritual practice. I finally had to admit that there was work to do on the emotional level, and that my growth will be limited until I do it, and that my particular discipline was unequipped to help me with this, beyond encouraging me to replace negative *feelings* with love.

I now see why the emotional level is so important. The emotional planes come before the spiritual. In our journey of consciousness, we must heal and clear the planes in ascending order: physical, emotional, mental, intellectual and spiritual.

Bypassing emotional healing will sabotage any healing. If we aim for the "spiritual" with no attention to *feelings*, we are bound to be unstable in our growth. We are likely to end up suppressing *feelings* in the name of spirituality, and the suppressed negative subconscious will continue to plague us.

In the healing community, another important realization about *feelings* has been emerging lately. More and more, we hear of the connection between suppressed *feelings* and poor health. Healing professionals are venturing the idea that in order to resolve health issues, we must resolve the emotional issues behind them. The awareness is growing that the unhealed, unreleased and trapped negative emotional energy keeps building inside and eventually manifests in the physical.

Achieve Vibrant Health

Contact the 3 healing energies of the universe.

Focus the healing energies into your body.

Heal and Release the suppressed psychic-emotional energy that results in disease

Understand how chronic conditions represent major Karmic life clearing missions and how to handle them.

How to handle pain so it results in Karmic clearing instead of merely suffering.

However, when I would read these statements in the past, I would usually be confused and disappointed. It was now clear to me that investigating and healing on the emotional level was something I had neglected and must do, **but** none of these spokespersons really had anything to offer in the way of actually how this might be accomplished, aside from the vague suggestion that *feelings* should be expressed instead of being held in.

What did express mean? Should I be more emotional? Should I lash out, should I hurt people who hurt me, should I yell and attack and get it off my chest? Should I be always out front and discuss all my *feelings*, or should I just get into therapy? And if so, what kind of therapy? Many of these possible alternatives clashed with higher principles that were now a part of my life. I *felt* that I was on my own.

Although emotional healing has always been an important goal of Western psychotherapy, this seemed like an incomplete answer for me. While I was sure that therapy could be helpful to certain people at certain times, in my situation it seemed a therapist was unwarranted - actually, I *felt* better than normal.

Therapy was also expensive and could only be undertaken for limited periods, and I was by no means convinced that it was the way to emotional well-being. Many of my friends who were in therapy were still greatly troubled by negative emotions. It's now apparent to me that most talk therapies never really touch *feelings*, something I have heard over and over in my counseling practice from clients who spent years in therapy.

What I wanted was an approach that I could use all the time, on my own. It was also important for me to integrate my emotional healing with my consciousness investigating and healing. How to do this in traditional therapy? Seeing no clear direction, I decided that I must break new ground.

It's still 1988. I'm intently searching for a way to put this together. I come into contact with a teacher who seems to be presenting Eastern philosophy in a new way. I already know a lot about Eastern philosophy, **but** all of what I had been exposed to was *old school*, if I may use that term.

The old school never really recognized negative *feelings* - just be spiritual, it said. If you *felt* angry, be loving. In other words, suppress your anger. This new teacher had things to say that I had never heard. Maybe I was just never ready to hear before now, **but** the revolution was beginning within me.

I started having tremendous insights. I realized that a large part of how I saw the world and how I experienced my interactions with others was based on projection. In projection, it would appear that someone or something was responsible for my experience. In other words, I believed that someone or something was making me angry, lonely, afraid, hateful, depressed and so on.

What I realized was that these *feelings* were actually coming from my suppressed emotional subconscious and just attaching to people and circumstances outside myself. Taking it a step further, I could see how I attracted difficult people and circumstances to myself that corresponded to the *feelings*. Why would I do this, I asked? The answer came that it was in order to bring up the suppressed *feelings* for healing, transmuting and clearing.

A Large Light Went On.

You mean I attract these difficult people and situations to myself in order to bring up those suppressed, negative *feelings* from my subconscious for healing and clearing? Yes, the answer came.

And if I miss taking advantage of this opportunity to heal and clear the *feelings*, I'll continue to attract this same type of person and circumstance to myself, over and over? Yes, the answer came.

This is starting to sound something like Karma. Yes, the answer came.

I was stunned.

For the first time, I saw the connection between the Karma of the East and the suppressed emotional subconscious of the West. For the first time, I saw the complete implication and importance of taking responsibility for my emotional experience. And at the same time how I never took responsibility! How I would blame, blame, blame, and unconsciously blame more.

The Emotional Clearing Process

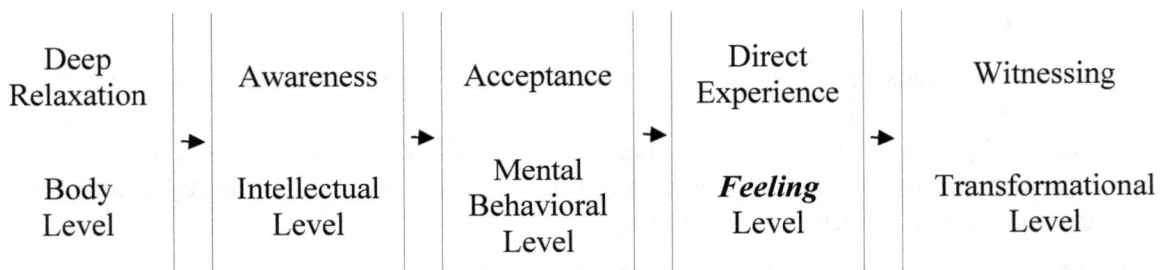

Deep Relaxation		Awareness		Acceptance		Direct Experience		Witnessing
Body Level	→	Intellectual Level	→	Mental Behavioral Level	→	*Feeling* Level	→	Transformational Level

As the fog lifted and what was to become the *Emotional Clearing Process* started to come together in my brain, I saw that the first step to healing my emotional self was the meditative state or Deep Relaxation. I naturally started to use breath and body techniques that I had learned in my Yoga practice to facilitate Deep Relaxation, even incorporating Binaural Beat Technology to help induce Alpha.

1. Deep Relaxation

In Deep Relaxation, brainwaves slow down to the Alpha level (8-13 cps) or deeper. This corresponds to a quieting of left-brain, ego-based activity: Thinking, reasoning, planning, judging, worrying, and above all, doing, diminish. Consciousness starts to shift to the right-brain, the seat of authentic *feeling*.

The right-brain Alpha state is essential for emotional healing. The quieting of the left-brain mind allows you to operate on the *feeling* level, accessing and releasing the deep, hidden, core *feelings* that are behind the painful events you draw to yourself.

2. Awareness

After Relaxation, the next step is Awareness. This consists of several parts:

    1. Become aware of the *feeling* behind the event.

2. Understand how the *feeling* is coming from the suppressed, unconscious reservoir within, and is only being triggered by and projected **onto** the event, even attracting it to you.

3. Take responsibility for the *feeling*.

At this point, I saw my experience in a completely new way, **but** I still needed to learn how to go about handling *feelings* instead of suppressing them and how to heal and release already suppressed *feelings* as they came up for clearing.

Gradually, the light grew brighter. I saw that all we need to do is to experience *feelings* fully as they occur in order to heal, transmute and release the negative *feelings* and to integrate the positive.

We think we are experiencing our *feelings*, **but** the problem is that we avoid allowing full *feeling* to occur; in fact, it is reasonable to assert that in today's world, most of us have actually lost the capacity for authentic *feeling*.

Rebuilding The Capacity For Authentic *Feeling*

If full *feeling* occurs, the *feeling* energy is exhausted, and no suppression takes place. *Feelings* that have been suppressed must be brought into awareness and experienced to heal, transmute and clear them There are ways to do this that make it peaceful, even joyful, instead of something to be dreaded.

The remedy for suppression is to experience the *feeling*. Expression without *feelings* is ineffective

It's our unconscious inner resistance to the *feeling* that blocks it from coming fully into consciousness so it can heal and release spontaneously. We resist painful *feelings* instinctively, **but** we must learn that resistance is usually out of harmony with our best interest.

Resistance itself constitutes most of the pain associated with any distressful emotional event.

If we can drop resistance, and open completely to the *feeling*, pain immediately lessens and healing and clearing occurs, and we regain our *feeling* capacity.

3. Acceptance

I saw that the next step would be Acceptance. Acceptance means opening to your *feelings* - dropping the inner resistance. Acceptance is different than accepting negative people or circumstances into your life. It refers primarily to your *feelings*, as they are, relative to the negative people or circumstances.

The inner resistance that blocks full *feeling* occurs on a mental level **but** it can take a certain behavioral form, which may need to be adjusted. For example, we can turn from the experience of pain by immersing ourselves in activity. We can use food, drugs, sex, entertainment as diversions from *feelings*. As we act out *feelings*, i.e., as we are motivated by *feelings* into taking action to change circumstances in order to change the *feeling*, we essentially close down to the full experience of the *feeling*.

More subtle forms of emotional avoidance are worrying, controlling, living in the past or future, living according to rigid concepts, judging self and others, even constantly seeking the answer or talking about the *feelings* instead of *feeling* them. And, of course, last **but** most popular, relationship dependencies. All these are addictions; ways of unconsciously **but** deliberately avoiding the *feelings*.

Overcome Addiction and Substance Abuse

Use with addictions to Alcohol, Drugs, Smoking, Food, Sex

Manage and transcend your addiction

Reduce cravings

Eliminate addictions by releasing the negative *feelings* behind them

Heal and Release psychological addictions to people, power, money and fame.

I realized that I had to train myself to weed out resistance and develop my capacity for *feeling*; and that in my quest for the past 20 years, I had been doing the exact opposite - pushing away *feelings* as I chased after happiness, wholeness, and "enlightenment."

4. Direct Experience

The next step is to move into what I call Direct Experience of the *feeling*. We have softened our resistances and now can access *feelings* more deeply. As I explored exactly how to do this, it came most naturally to me to use meditation as a format for exploring and experiencing *feelings*. Indeed, at this point, I regard the metaphysical tools of the East, such as meditation, 'breathwork', and 'bodywork' to be essential in this approach to healing and clearing *feelings*. When used with emotional healing and clearing as an intent, these tools greatly aid in both bringing up suppressed *feelings* and in the eventual healing and releasing.

In Direct Experience, you sit quietly and allow the conscious mind to come to rest. You can use any technique you may know to enter the stillness. You can just think of it as sitting quietly, doing nothing, if you happen to be allergic to that word meditation.

As you sit, *feelings* begin to emerge into your awareness. This is the releasing starting. The *feelings* are coming from the subconscious into conscious awareness for healing and clearing. Any negative *feeling* can come up, such as anxiety, fear, anger, sadness, rejection, heartbreak, humiliation, loneliness, hatred, inadequacy, frustrations or abuse of any sort including sexual and even depression.

If you sit and anger keeps jumping up from something that happened yesterday or ten years ago it means this *feeling* is coming up to be healed and cleared. Allow the *feeling* to be, allow it to exist on its own. Try to see if it has a place it your body. Breathe into it. Just watch and experience the *feeling*. Look at the *feeling* from the perspective of the first two steps: Take responsibility for the *feeling* - stop blaming and own it; look within for the subtle inner resistance to the *feeling* that keeps the *feeling* blocked and replace the resistance with acceptance, to whatever extent possible for you now.

Allow the *feeling* to come forward fully. There is no need to be afraid of it. Keep your attention on the breath - breathing easily and smoothly with a sense of breathing into the *feeling* and the body location to further loosen the congested energy of the *feeling*. As you sit and open to and experience the *feeling*, it is healing and clearing. Remain calm if the *feeling* becomes intense. Allow yourself to go through it. The experience will naturally wind down and you will *feel* a shift - you will have healed and released the *feeling* energy. It is possible you will have to repeat this at other times to completely heal and release the suppressed *feeling*, and important life "healing and clearing missions" may take years. Persevere and be patient, knowing and *feeling* that you are moving in the right direction.

Overcome Depression

Identify, heal and release the unconscious suppressed *feelings* that cause your depression.
Activate authentic self-esteem by accepting and honoring all parts of yourself, including your painful *feelings*.
Approach and reverse depression from an energetic viewpoint.

As I practiced truly experiencing my *feelings* instead of ignorantly avoiding them as I previously had, I began to *feel* that I was starting to come alive. It became apparent that the blocking of the negative *feelings* due my unconscious resistance also blocked my positive experience and expression of life. I *felt* myself really growing. Difficult situations changed magically because I no longer needed to attract them.

5. Witnessing

As I shared these insights with others, I was overjoyed to see them respond the same way. As I kept practicing, however, it seemed that one more step was needed. This last step is Witnessing. It is a deliberate move to invoke transcendental healing energies, and takes place on the spiritual level. Using this power greatly aids in the healing and clearing process.

Witnessing refers to a powerful shift of consciousness that awakens the transcendental spiritual energy in us, brings us into an Alpha healing state, and allows processing of difficult *feelings* to proceed easily. It means breaking the inner identification with the *feeling*; owning the *feeling*, **but** seeing it in a detached manner. It's a concrete, tangible experience of shifting from lower-self consciousness to higher-self consciousness.

When you're in the witness, you *feel* genuinely serene, peaceful, and accepting, no matter what's going on in your lower-self emotions. Therefore, establishing yourself in the witness is a preliminary to healing, transmuting and releasing negative *feelings*. You'll *feel* safe and confident as you approach *feelings*. If you ever *feel* yourself getting too much negative *feeling*, you just go back and reactivate the witness.

I have found the best way to awaken the witness and invoke transcendental healing energies in emotional processing is by utilizing the ancient Third Eye technique. At the very start of an *Emotional Clearing Process*, we contact the two Yin/Yang healing energies of the universe. Then we contact the transcendental witness by activating the Third Eye (on the forehead).

Activating the Third Eye achieves the same result as any of the *Rapid Eye Movement* therapies you may have heard about, except that it is more effective, and is the ancient, original technique. These other techniques were discovered accidentally and used because they worked. Activating the Third Eye chakra brings about an integration of left and right brains, and so reduces resistance to emotional experience, releasing the *feelings*, and you can do this without the help of a therapist if you want.

Make Your Relationship A Source Of Joy

Learn how to manage the *feelings* your relationship triggers.
Make your intimate relationship a vital part of your consciousness path.

Learn how to go beyond blaming your partner.

Transcend psychological dependency by recognizing and overcoming attachment.

As we take any *feeling* through these five steps, Deep Relaxation, Awareness, Acceptance, Direct Experience, and Witnessing, we are taking the *feeling* to a place where healing, transmutation, releasing and integrating can occur. Trying to apply any of the steps without the others is less effective.

The Process of Entering The Witness

If you are sensitive or if you have been practicing, the first three steps will have brought you at least partially into alpha. This last step will bring you all the way.

Witnessing is vital in processing. *Witnessing provides the power and perspective to confront the strong negative energies that are surfacing.* The Witness is the key inner orientation for processing *feelings*. It gives you the ability to detach from negativity without being overcome by it.

As you practice, you will gain an appreciation of what the Witness *feels* like. It is a sense of being detached from whatever is going on around you or inside you and at the same time also sensing your connection to it on a deeper level. Your sense of physical perspective may change. You *feel* the healing power and joy of self-love. When you have become familiar with the sensation of being in the Witness, you will know when you have to reactivate it in order to maintain the sense of *disidentification* that is so important when healing, transmuting and releasing lower chakra *feelings*, even if they are coming from a higher level. After you become proficient, you will be able to activate the Witness in seconds or less. Just remembering to do it will be enough. Witness consciousness can be entered during activity as well as meditation; maintaining the Witness during activity will become second nature.

Activating Healing Energy By Entering The Witness
The Actual Process

1. Breath Relaxation (Blocks in the breath reflect blocks in the chakras) (about 2 minutes)

Feel the connection to your body. Allow yourself to come into the moment, through sensing your connection to the body. Drop all sense of striving. Drop all intention to achieve anything, even in these exercises. Come more and more into the moment, the place where healing occurs and where the Witness resides. Begin a gentle connected breath, with a 1:1 ratio of inhale to exhale. Breathe easily and smoothly. Watch the breath as it comes in and goes out. *Feel* it in the body. Again drop all sense of striving, of needing to make anything happen. Allow everything to be as it is. Gently keep breathing, with the conscious connection of inhale and exhale. Allow the breath to take you to deep alpha levels of relaxation and quiet in the body.

2. Aura Strengthening (about 2 to 5 minutes, maybe less)

Continue the connected breath without paying attention to it. Let it find its own level. Visualize your aura around you. See a sphere approximately six feet in diameter with colorful, charged electrical particles inside. As you inhale, visualize a beam of luminescent, silver-white light shining down from the sun, entering the top of your head, and going down to your solar plexus, where it forms an energy ball about one foot in diameter. See the light as dazzling and powerful; burning away any negativity it encounters. As you exhale, visualize the energy ball at your solar plexus expanding outward to fill the entire space inside your aura. Visualize the particles extending to the edge of your aura, where they form a shell. Visualize (see and *feel*) the shell as strong and impenetrable. Visualize vibrations outside the shell being deflected as they try to pass through. See your energy inside being retained. *Feel* deeply the archetypal, yang, masculine qualities of the light, and your relation to them: strength, protection, assertiveness, will, competence.

3. Grounding (about 2 to 5 minutes, maybe less)

Continue the connected breath. Remember to both see and *feel* as you visualize. Visualize an earth link from the center of the earth **to** your 'Survival Center', located at the base of the spine (same place as the first chakra). As you inhale, visualize blue-green earth energy coming from the center of the earth along the link, touching your 'Survival Center', and filling up your entire body. Experience the energy as vibrant, warm, nurturing, loving. Visualize/Create a second earth link; **from** your 'Survival Center', located at the base of the spine (same place as the first chakra), back to the center of the earth and all her selves. As you exhale, visualize the blue-green color of the second earth link absorbing negativity, turning to a reddish-black color, and being pulled by the earth through the 'Survival Center' (at the first chakra), back to the center of the earth, where it is transmuted and neutralized. See it being neutralized and dissolving into the earth. Invoke the presence of the archetypal, yin, feminine by simply inviting her. Allow the qualities of the feminine to come forward, and *feel* them deeply: softness, caring, receptivity, compassion, nurturing, sensuality, unconditional love

4. Entering The Witness (about 2 to 15 minutes, maybe less)

Continue the same breath. Keeping your eyes closed, look up with the physical eyes to the Third Eye point. This point is between and above the eyebrows, on the forehead. Strain the eyes slightly, looking up as far as possible. Look into the blackness with the physical eyes. Keep straining as long as comfortable – it is the straining that activates the psycho-physiological response.

Visualize both yang (masculine) energy coming from above and yin (feminine) energy coming from below, meeting at the Third Eye as you inhale. As you exhale, visualize the energies spinning clockwise or just being still in the Third Eye, whichever *feels* best. You may want to use only one of these energies, depending on which you need most.

Invite the Witness to come forward. *Feel* the qualities of the Witness: detachment from the Lower Self body, detachment from thoughts, and detachment from *feelings*; disidentification; choicelessness; unconditional happiness.

Just sitting still gives the subconscious the opportunity to bring its suppressed contents to consciousness. Allow the *feelings* just to be.

A suppressed *feeling* will come up. This occurrence is distinguished by the emergence of emotion, sometimes strong. This is what you want. Recognize that healing and clearing is happening. Stay with the *feeling* and with any associated thoughts or images, such as interaction with another person, group or situation. Move into a processing mode – own (welcome), accept, experience, witness, process and allow the *feeling*/emotion to heal, transmute, release and integrate. Allow the *feeling* to remain in your consciousness until you *feel* a shift – until the *feeling* starts to link to another related *feeling* or diminishes/dissolves..

5. Closing

Ground down to the earth one final time through the second earth link **from** your 'Survival Center' to earth and disperse all negativity. See the negativity being absorbed and neutralized/transmuted by the earth.

and at the same time

Bring in more white light from above for yourself and all of Earths selves and more blue-green earth energy coming from the center of the earth along the first earth link, touching your 'Survival Center', and filling up your entire body. Experience the energy as vibrant, warm, nurturing, loving. *Feel* it as joyous and powerful, filling any dark places that have resulted from negativity releasing.

6. When you are done you may open your eyes.

Adapted by author from additional pages of <http://www.emclear.com/>

Chapter 13
Self Reflection And Questions To Ask Yourself
The Importance Of The Subconscious Mind As A Key

Unihipili: *(u·hi·ni·pi·li)* is the Hawaiian name for what is sometimes called the subconscious /inner/emotional/intuitive mind. I use the name 'Unihipili' because there is nothing sub about the subconscious mind. It may need our LOVE and guidance; however, in many, and probably in most ways, it is much more powerful than the conscious mind. Even though the Unihipili is much more powerful than the conscious mind, it is in many ways like a three or four year old child. It needs guidance and LOVE. It also likes to investigate. The Unihipili, or child within, will respond or react according to your "choice". The Unihipili, like children, dislikes work and likes to play. Therefore I use the word *work* carefully when doing any kind of healing, transmuting, releasing and integrating.

To heal and clear myself, I primarily use the ways explained in this book and in my first book, *Two Choices: Divine LOVE Or Anything Else.* Use whatever ways *feel* right for you.

While Using The Tables Below As A Guide:

1) When you make a statement or ask a question you may get a strong *feeling* or a more subtle *feeling*. If you wish, you can indicate the strength. Remember there are no 'right' or 'wrong' answers, only a chance to shed light on your beliefs. The statements in the following sections are questions made as statements to help get *feeling*s without waiting for or needing yes/no answers.

2) Sometime you may get a *feeling* of neutrality or no *feeling*. You can also indicate that. Notice if you get a good relaxed *feeling* or a constricted or unpleasant *feeling* before you even finish the statement. This *feeling* is from your subconscious mind (Unihipili) before you have a chance to analyze or intellectualize. Allow the flow **and then** analyze if you *feel* the need.

3) Use your increased awareness and intuition to investigate and heal as you wish.

4) Follow the sections below in order and realize that after you have investigated, healed, transmuted, released and integrated at each section you may want to go through them in order several times. As your clarity and awareness increase, you will be able to heal more each time. This is an ongoing journey.

The first twelve sections of this chapter are inspired by and based on the book, *Everyday Enlightenment - The Twelve Gateways to Personal Growth* by Dan Millman. There are twelve sections or categories closely based on what Dan Millman calls 'gateways'. I prefer to allow you to decide for yourself how to think of them and what to call them.

I was taught to make all questions into statements because the universe only understand yes or no. I realized if the statement is a negative, saying it as a statement can sometimes energize the negative. I have reworded statements into questions with yes or no answers to avoid inadvertently energizing a negative. Avoid the using the words *not, n't, but* and *however* in your questions. Use simple, single, questions that can be answered with a yes or no.

Turn the question over to Great Spirit/God/Divinity and your Higher Self without attachment to a desired outcome or an expectation. Allow the answer to come from them.

1 – Worthiness

The central premise of this first section is that our sense of self-worth is the single most important determinant of the health, abundance and joy we allow into our lives. Discover your self-worth. It is already here and needs to be accepted. You get only what you **believe** you deserve; no more and no less. We **subconsciously** choose or attract into our lives those people and experiences we believe we deserve (Are Worthy Of).

Worthiness - Statements/Questions	Best If	Before Clearing	After Clearing
Do I believe there is a need to be worthy in order to attract and accept 'good'?	NO		
Do I feel unworthy?	NO		
Do I *feel* deserving of 'good'?	YES		
Do I feel that I am worthy?	YES		
Do I feel totally worthy?	YES		
Have I transcended the need for self-worth and am I simply willing to accept life's blessings and opportunities no matter what my *feelings* of self-worth?	YES		
Repeat the same questions using your full birth name and any other name you go by instead of 'I'			

Personal Notes

2- Reclaim Your Will

Three Magic words; "Just Do It". Assert your power to act upon what you know and *feel*. Everything is easier said than done until you do it. No matter how talented or intelligent you are, it is your thoughts and actions that shape your destiny

Prayer, affirmations, meditation, mantras, sound healing, etc all have their place. Remember you are responsible to do your part. If you sit on the couch and eat or drink all day and say affirmations, do mantras and pray, "make me healthy" or "make me wealthy", do you really expect to be made healthy or wealthy. If you go to seminars, retreats and gatherings without taking responsibility and action for yourself, why go?

I am slightly overweight and out of shape. (Silent "Cancel/Clear"). Reworded to "I choose to lose some weight and get in better shape." How do I do it? Start by "Reclaiming My Will" and "Energizing My Body".

It takes more than will power and "Just Do It" to make a journey. You need a direction. Set priorities.

When you have difficulty completing a task or reaching a goal, it may be something other than a lack of will. It may be self-doubt, fear of failure or ridicule, lack of planning or lack of focus.

Keep it simple and fun so what you do becomes a positive and fun action for you and your subconscious mind (Unihipili).

In any challenging situation ask yourself, "What would my strongest, bravest, most courageous most loving part do right now?" Then do it

Reclaim Your Will - Statements/Questions	Best If	Before Clearing	After Clearing
Do I turn what I know and want to do into what I do?	YES		
Do I apply my will to eating healthier?	YES		
Do I apply my will to exercise adequately, appropriately and properly?	YES		
Do I apply my will to my budget and finances in order to prosper?	YES		
Do I apply my will to act with kindness or courtesy even when I *feel* unkind, impatient or *feel* like being rude?	YES		
Have I committed to "Reclaim My Will" and do I have a simple routine in place that I can follow each day in order to (plan _____)?	YES		
Have I "Reclaimed My Will?	YES		
What is my goal this minute? (_____)			
What is my goal this hour? (_____)			
What is my goal this week? (_____)			
What is my goal this month? (_____)			
What is my goal this year? (_____)			
Repeat the same questions using your full birth name and any other name you go by instead of 'I'			

3 – Energize Your Body

Your body is the only thing you are guaranteed to keep for an entire lifetime. The human journey begins and ends with the body.

Even now, abundant energy flows through the world, swirling around you, flowing through you. Your primary task in managing energy is to clear internal energy leaks and blockages so you can maintain a higher energy level.

Energy leaks and blockages can stem from mental sources (including anxiety, worry, regret and preoccupation), emotional sources (including fear, sorrow and anger), or physical sources (including illness, injuries, postural imbalances and overloaded digestive systems). All of these produce tension and discomfort, which reduce physical vitality.

To understand how and why you have developed energy leaks and blockages, imagine a flowing river whose water represents the energy flowing through your body. A free-flowing river has great energy and power. If trees or boulders obstruct the flow, it creates turbulence, restricts the natural flow and creates side channels where some of the water (energy) is misplaced. In your body you experience these obstructions, this turbulence, as tension and discomfort, which in turn drain your energy and may lead to disease.

Take one slow, deep breath - as slowly and deeply as you can comfortably, expanding first your belly and then your chest. *Feel* yourself relax as you exhale slowly. Make it a habit to do this at least once each hour throughout the day.

Remember to eat well, exercise in some way regularly and get enough rest.

When your body experiences tension, discomfort or pain it may be caused by energy blockages. There are two primary ways to reduce the discomfort.

1) You can clear the mental, emotional and physical blockages, which can be done in many

   ways, some of which are explained in this book. This allows energy to flow as intended.

2) You can lower the level of energy in your body. The most common forms of tension

   (energy) release according to Dan Millman are exercise, sexual climax, creative endeavors, physical and mental overexertion, thrill seeking (including gambling, suspense films and video games), overeating and the use of alcohol or other drugs. These all can be a repetitive cycles known as addiction.

Dan Millman suggests to start each and every morning with one jumping jack as a start. You may want to start by stretching your back while lying on the floor for 20 seconds, followed by a 10 second leg lift and 1 sit up. What can you commit to comfortably and safely and "Just Do It" in order to begin the process of reclaiming you will.

Energize Your Body - Statements/Questions	Best If	Before Clearing	After Clearing
Do I normally eat well.?	YES		
Do I normally exercise regularly and adequately?	YES		
Do I normally get enough rest and sleep.?	YES		
Am I energizing my body by (exercising)) each day?	YES		
Am I energizing my body by (eating healthy) each day?	YES		
Am I energizing my body by (_____) each day?			
Am I clearing the mental, emotional and physical blockages and allowing energy flow as intended by (_____)?			
Am I clearing the mental, emotional and physical blockages and allowing energy flow as intended by (_____)?			
Am I clearing the mental, emotional and physical blockages and allowing energy flow as intended by (_____)?			
Am I releasing excess energy in a healthful positive manner by (_____)?			
Am I releasing excess energy in a healthful positive manner by (_____)?			
Am I releasing excess energy in a healthful positive manner by (_____)?			
Repeat the same questions using your full birth name and any other name you go by instead of 'I'			

4 – Money And Abundance

When you know you have a negative or limiting belief about money and abundance, you are free to examine it, heal it and release it if you choose. No such choice exists for unconscious beliefs or unexamined attitudes.

Money and Abundance - Statements/Questions	Best If	Before Clearing	After Clearing
Do I have judgment towards money?	NO		
Do I have mixed, negative or judgmental *feelings* about people like Deepak Chopra or healers/teachers who posses money in abundance and have houses valued in the millions?	NO		
Do I have mixed, negative or judgmental *feelings* about people like actors and athletes who posses money in abundance and have houses valued in the millions?	NO		
Do I have mixed, negative or judgmental *feelings* about people who are insensitive, uncaring and dismissive towards those in need?	NO		
Do I have a *feeling* of guilt that keeps me from having money in abundance myself?	NO		
Do I associate Poverty with humility, goodness and spirituality.?	NO		
Do I associate wealth with greed, badness and arrogance?	NO		
Do I associate poverty with virtue?	NO		
Do I associate wealth with 'sin'?	NO		
Do I have an aversion to having my own money in abundance and being wealthy?	NO		
Do I have a fear of having my own money in abundance and being wealthy?	NO		
Do I believe that true teachers should expect nothing for their teachings except gratitude and thanks?	NO		
Do I feel it will help others if I remain poor?	NO		
Do I confuse the idea of letting go of attachments with giving away all my earthly goods?	NO		
Do I clearly see my negative and limiting beliefs about having my own money in abundance and being wealthy?	YES		
Have I honestly examined my values, beliefs and inner hurdles that stand between me and self sufficiency, having my own money in abundance and my being wealthy?	YES		
Have I examined and healed, transmuted and released all my negative or limiting beliefs about money and abundance?	YES		
Am I willing and ready to attract, accept and enjoy abundance, wealth and respect?	YES		
Do I gratefully and openly accept gifts for my sharing?	YES		
Do I recognize and accept that times have changed and money, if freely given, is the same as accepting food, shelter, moccasins, a chicken or any other gift for my sharing.	YES		

Do I know and am aware that free exchange of gifts, including money, is part of the Divine Plan and Divine Flow.	YES		
If I had enough money to live on for the rest of my life and money was no concern what would I be doing at this exact moment?			
If I had enough money to live on for the rest of my life what would I do with my time? (When you have the answer find work in the area if you can.)			
Repeat the same questions using your full birth name and any other name you go by instead of 'I'			

Give and accept thanks with LOVE. You may find yourself saying "thank you, your welcome" to more and more people. There is always an exchange.

5 – Tame Your Mind

You can no more control or quiet your thoughts in any lasting way than you can stop the weather. You can control your response to them.

Let your thoughts be whatever they are, positive or negative, and get on with your life. Learn self-compassion; make peace with your mind.

Thoughts arise of their own accord from the subconscious mind (Unihipili) in a subliminal flow. Sometimes they get your conscious attention (you notice that you are thinking thoughts); mostly they pass unnoticed, like a subconscious stream. These thoughts manifest as subliminal whispers, becoming moods, emotions, desires, and impulses. When unnoticed, they operate like hypnotic suggestions to influence your behavior. When you observe them consciously as thoughts (as you do in meditation), a healing takes place, because thoughts, fears, beliefs, and associations are clarified in the light of awareness, lose their power to distort your reality, control your moods or limit your life.

Meditation can become a moment to moment practice of daily life, without the need for any special setting or position

Tame Your Mind - Statements/Questions	Best If	Before Clearing	After Clearing
Do I try to tame my mind by trying to subjugate, control or quiet it?	NO		
Do I tame my mind by making peace with it and my thoughts?	YES		
Do I examine my subconscious in order to heal, transmute, release and integrate the positive aspects of what I have considered bad or negative?	YES		
Do I listen to my intuition without interference of my conscious analyzing mind and without subjective filters?	YES		
Do I combine my intuition and logic as is best	YES		
Repeat the same questions using your full birth name and any other name you go by instead of 'I'			

6 – Trust Your Intuition

There is a difference between 'brain' and 'mind'. Our brain is a physical part of our physical body. Our mind is much more. Our brain does have two hemispheres. The left brain deals with logic and data and the right brain deals with *feeling*s, emotions and intuition. This is an oversimplification and some processes spread across the divide. The right brain is the part of the brain that connects with mind. Mind may be unlimited and includes:

Aumakua: (*au·ma·ku·a*)
The Hawaiian name for what is sometimes called the super-conscious/connection with the divine.
It is also defined as Hawaiian Ancestral Spirits.

Unihipili: (*u·hi·ni·pi·li*)
The Hawaiian name for what is sometimes called the subconscious /inner/emotional/intuitive mind. I use the name 'Unihipili' because there is nothing sub about the subconscious. It may need our LOVE and guidance; however, in many, and probably in most ways, it is much more powerful than the conscious mind.

Uhane: (*u·ha·ne*)
The Hawaiian name for what is sometimes called the consciousness/waking/rational mind.

Logic interferes with intuition and *feeling*. Use them both, at different times. Let go of logic when accessing intuition. Allow intuition to supplement and improve logic.

Intuition is different than what most people think it is; in fact, it is totally different than thinking. Reason may complement or interfere with intuition. There is no substitute for intuition. Intuition comes from a different side of the brain and source than logic. Everyday enlightenment requires full use of both sides of our brains, integrating the logical and the intuitive, the conscious mind and the subconscious mind (Unihipili), science and mysticism, to form a full representation of reality

Intuitive *feelings* are related to and different from emotional *feeling*. Someone out of touch with their emotions is usually out of touch with their intuitive *feelings* as well. Intuition is *feeling* - impression or sensation that can also arise as what we call "funny *feeling*" or in the form of images, sounds, and (on rare occasions) taste or smell. Instinct is more closely identified as a gut-level sensation, intuition is often a non-localized impression or *feeling*. Instinct and intuition are both related to right-brain capacities and the subconscious mind (Unihipili).

When you understand the ordinary rather than magical nature of intuition, you begin to trust your innate ability to know without knowing how. The factors we weigh in making logical decisions are only the proverbial tip of the iceberg. Our subconscious mind (Unihipili) also accesses what is below "see" level where there are variables our conscious, thinking, mind is unaware of. So intuitive decisions tend to be more aligned with our subconscious mission and destiny of which our conscious reasoning mind is unaware.

Trust Your Intuition - Statements/Questions	Best If	Before Clearing	After Clearing
Do I place more faith in the guidance and intuition of others than I do my own?	NO		
Do I distrust my intuition.?	NO		
If someone offers guidance that conflicts with or disagrees with my intuition and guidance do I trust my guidance more?	YES		
Do I know what intuition is?	YES		
Do I usually trust my intuition?	YES		
Do I trust *my* intuition rather than relying on the intuitive skills of others?	YES		
Do I trust *my* intuition above all others?	YES		
Do I always trust my intuition?	Best If YES		
Repeat the same questions using your full birth name and any other name you go by instead of 'I'			

7 - Accept Your *Feelings* And Emotions

In polite society we are taught to hide and rarely show many strong emotions, almost as if they are non-existent. Up until now, most people have followed this teaching without realizing it. Emotions are as natural to humans as breathing. By hiding our *feelings* and emotions we end up suppressing them, losing touch with them and getting sick. Sometimes, as the pressure builds, we experience emotional episodes such as arguments or explosions (and we may later berate ourselves for having "lost control").

The day you were told that big boys (or girls) "do**n't** cry", the first time someone asked you *why* you were upset, the day you learned that you upset others when you expressed your anger, you began to cut yourself off from accepting (or even recognizing) your own *feelings*. You learned to intellectualize your emotions and started to analyze, suppress, justify, and deny them. Your exile from the Garden of Emotional Authenticity had begun.

When we devalue or deny our emotional energies, we pay a physical price. Chronic emotional tension can generate or aggravate symptoms such as headaches, backaches, arthritis, hypertension and high blood pressure, dyspepsia, colitis. It aggravates conditions such as ulcers and insomnia, and other psychosomatic ailments. And as we age, tension produced from holding in unexpressed emotions tends to produce physical stiffness, muscle aches and pains, and reduced flexibility. Movement becomes more painful, so we move less, thereby reducing our range of movement, our range of life. In some elderly people you can see the cumulative effect of denied emotions stored as chronic tension. Such restriction can even create a mental condition called "psychosclerosis" - hardening of the attitudes. Psychologist Wilhelm Reich would remind his clients that unexplored and unhealed emotions are stored in the flexor muscles of the body, and the organs weep the tears that the eyes refuse to shed.

Those of us most out of touch with our emotions are usually also out of touch with our bodies. When athletes ignore physical pain, this may have short-term benefits. In the long term, when athletes play through physical pain and injuries they may have ongoing problems for the rest of their lives. The same is true for tuning out our *feelings*. When we lose emotional sensitivity we also lose touch with our intuitive capacities.

In losing touch with our *feelings*, we also lose touch with the *feelings* of others. It can come to the point that we live in a kind of benumbed state, *feeling* disconnected or dissociated from life. In fact, what some of us have experienced as a spiritual problem (a sense of disconnection from God/Great Spirit) is actually an emotional problem (a disconnection from *feeling*).

If you are unsure what you *feel* - whether you are afraid or hurt or angry - the following exercise can help attune your emotional awareness and, in the process, improve your intuitive capacities and empathy in relationships.

When you think you may be upset and are unclear about what you *feel*, ask yourself, "If I *felt* something right now, would it be closer to fear, sorrow, or anger?"

You may respond, "I do**n't** know how I *feel*." Persist with yourself. "If I knew - if I suddenly had an insight, or if the *feeling* became so strong it was obvious - would it be closer to fear, sorrow, or anger?"

Then make a statement to yourself or to another. "I *feel* (_____). "
This is a first step toward reintegrating your *feelings* into your body and your life and opening deeper levels of authenticity. It is important to say "I *feel*" instead of "I am".

Again, to accept your emotions, you have to know them. Of the two levels of emotional authenticity - knowing your *feelings* and expressing them - knowing is the most important. You always want to know what you *feel*, Sometimes it is best to leave the *feelings* unexpressed. Sometimes we *feel* better when we get something off our chest - and sometimes we *feel* worse. That's why there is no hard and-fast rule about expressing what you *feel*. Always acknowledge your *feelings*, at least to yourself, to avoid suppressing them and having them become hidden and trapped.

Expressing your *feelings* can be an act of courage and honesty that provides valuable feedback to others who may be unaware the impact their words or deeds have. Remaining silent out of politeness, stoicism or discomfort is a disservice to yourself and others, and only creates more turmoil. Expressing yourself in a blaming manner also creates more turmoil without resolution: "You messed up again! You make me so angry, you jerk!"

Expressing your truth in a **respectful way** makes it more likely to be heard. Realize that your truth is based on your beliefs and perceptions.

Skillful expression means sometimes using "I" words rather than "you" words. Three examples follow.

"When you say (or do) (_____), I *feel* (_____)".

"**I would** appreciate it if you would say (or do) (_____)
instead of" (_____)".

"**I have** a hard time being around you when you act like (_____)"."

That way you've defined your boundaries and expressed your *feelings*. Leave it at that. No need to criticize, patronize, ostracize or justify.

You can deliver any message if it's in the right envelope - and has a return address. If you get a response, just listen.

The ability to express *feelings* is an important life skill. Forever expressing upset *feelings* tends to re-stimulate them. Learn to stand up for yourself and define clear boundaries, without centering your life around the never-ending cycle of *feel* and express or constantly checking out your sensitivities, looking to see if anyone has offended you. There is no need for other people to hear about every *feeling* you have. Find a constructive balance.

Accept Your *Feelings* and Emotions - Statements/Questions	Best If	Before Clearing	After Clearing
Do I sometimes suppress my *feelings* or emotions?	NO		
Is it ok to **act** on **any** feeling or emotion even if hurtful or negative?	NO		
When I *feel* anger, jealousy, judgment, fear or hatred do I hold onto the feeling and let it affect me?	NO		
Do I accept my *feelings* and emotions with unconditional LOVE and acceptance?	YES		
When I *feel* anger, jealousy, judgment, fear or hatred, do I heal, LOVE, clear and release it?	YES		
Is it is ok to *feel* **anything**?	YES		
Do I choose to *feel* and be LOVING instead of feeling angry?	YES		
Repeat the same questions using your full birth name and any other name you go by instead of 'I'			

Personal Notes

8- Face Your Fears and Feelings

This section (what Dan Millman calls a gateway) could have come first. It is eighth because fear can be so intimidating an adversary, that you need the power of the previous 'gateways' to prepare for this 'gateway'.

Whatever the sources of fear, if you run from it you limit yourself. Many of us avoid emotional confrontations rather than staying present and resolving them.

It is natural and even appropriate - even a sign of sanity - to let fear guide you in physically dangerous situations where a lack of attention or care could mean injury or death.

Fear begins as a thought, *feeling*, belief, or expectation and it ends up stored in your body as physical tension and inhibited or shallow breathing unless you deal with it. There are many ways do deal with fear. Some ways of dealing with fear are to work directly with the body through massage, stretching and deep breathing. Other ways are through some form of energy work such as hypnosis, healing and releasing trapped and suppressed *feelings* and emotions.

Physical fears are direct, objective and realistic. In the unlikely event that something goes wrong when you are skydiving, you may receive an injury or may even die. Fear advises that you take precautions.

Psychological fears are indirect, subjective, and symbolic. The sky stays in place if you forget a speech or sing off-key or fail an exam - there is no risk of physical injury or death. If you go deeper into your psyche, you'll find that you are afraid of what failure represents instead of failure itself: issues of psychological survival, primal fears of losing face, of rejection, abandonment, ostracism, worthlessness, and mediocrity, of being a charlatan and a fool.

We often say "I ca**n't**" when what we really mean is "I do**n't** want to" or "I wo**n't**".

Phobia is a fancy psychological name for a big fear. Little fears generate subtle physiological reactions; big fears generate dramatic ones. When our physiological reactions to elevators, closets, wide-open spaces, dogs, cats, snakes, spiders, mice, moths or other insects or heights become unpleasant enough, we call them phobias.

Do you have any phobias?

What are your five worst fears? Failure? Losing face (shame, embarrassment, ridicule)? Rejection? Inadequacy or mediocrity? Public speaking? Pain? Heights? Insects? Animal(s)? Enclosed spaces? People?

If you could save the life of a child by doing what you most fear, would you?

As you overcome your fears, in what specific ways might your life change?

The deeper your understanding, the greater your power. As awareness penetrates a fear, it starts to dissolve fear at its core. Many of us misunderstand the nature of fear and of courage.

Chronic fear-produced muscular tension limits movement patterns, causing physical pain or even biological anesthesia (blocked sensation). We begin to restrict ways of moving and thinking, losing degrees of awareness, cleverness, spontaneity, and other cerebral functions. Take direct responsibility for clearing the fear-produced tension in our own bodies. By working gently, deeply, respectfully, into each area of stored tension, we produce a more vital, elastic and youthful body. Use both energetic and physical methods as appropriate.

Face Your Fears - Statements/Questions	Best If	Before Clearing	After Clearing
Do I sometimes avoid trying anything new to avoid *feeling* incompetent or appearing foolish or silly?	NO		
Do I avoid fully committing to an effort so that I can console myself with thoughts such as "If I had really tried, I could have done it."?	NO		
Do I avoid, whenever possible, any situation in which someone else has control. because of the fear of being out of control?	NO		
Do I sometimes hold myself back from achieving success out of the fear that success will leave me unfulfilled or with nothing left to do?	NO		
Do I sometimes avoid expressing my true *feelings* out of fear that the *feelings* may come back to me and cause discomfort?	NO		
Do I sometimes give myself a label that becomes both explanation and excuse: An example is, " I have a phobia about (_____) and therefore it is beyond me."?	NO		
Am I sometimes timid, shy, insecure, or suffering because of self-doubt?	NO		
Do I fear opening my heart.?	NO		
Do I fear vulnerability through the achievement of success?	NO		
Do I know that the expression of vulnerability can be my greatest gift and strength?	YES		
Do I have at least one habit that acts as a block in order to avoid facing my fears and feelings?	YES or NO		
If so, what is the habit and what is it blocking. (_____)			
Repeat the same questions using your full birth name and any other name you go by instead of 'I'			

9 - Illuminate Your Shadow

The shadow is the sum of those aspects of your being that you denied, devalued, and disowned. In other words, your shadow is what you insist you are **not**.

Imagine a great wolf-dog you bring home one day, whom others in your household disapprove of, so that you come to disapprove of him yourself and lock him down in the basement. The wolf-dog has qualities of loyalty, courage and sensitivity. It can also be menacing, ferocious and dangerous if left unloved or mistreated . You tell the others he is gone; you deny he lives there anymore. After a while you begin to forget he exists. He is there, growing more ferocious and menacing. If only you brought him out into the sunlight, stood up for him, let him run and play and use his power to pull your sled through the snow, to protect the household. In denying him, you lose his positive qualities. One day he may even break free from the basement, a ravening and destructive beast, or so a part of your fears. Remember, he is only an abandoned wolf-dog of many qualities, locked in the basement.

Your personal shadow consists of all those qualities you deny, repress, suppress and believe to be evil, immoral, abnormal or negative - the dust you sweep under the rug of your awareness and disown.

If you are raised in a pacifist household, you may reject your assertive side. In contrast, if you are raised in a highly competitive household, you may reject your gentle, sensitive side. What you reject, for whatever reason, becomes part of your shadow.

In fact, your shadow also contains potentially positive qualities. Many men, rejecting fear, push their sensitive, nourishing, childlike qualities into their shadow. Many women, reject anger and push assertive warrior qualities into their shadow. Antisocial individuals act out qualities society rejects, while denying their fearful, confused, vulnerable, even compassionate qualities, believing they represent weaknesses.

Everything contains its opposite. Clowns and comedians have a sad, cynical side; sweet people have a sour shadow; inside a pessimist you find a hopeful optimist; scratch a puritan and just beneath the surface there's a raving hedonist, begging for sex and chocolate. The truth of the shadow is this: You contain all things - highs and lows, saint and sinner, moralist and libertine.

Illuminating your shadow is different than inviting the devil to dinner or allowing your negative qualities or impulses to influence your behavior. When you have seen your dark side, you can make a clearer choice about how you will behave. Knowing that I have a lazy side helps me to consciously apply myself to my work rather than give in to my tendency to avoid exertion.

For some of us, personal growth has become a never-ending self improvement program - working to develop a nicer, happier, more secure personality. Many of us with low self-esteem *feel* insecure because we have based our esteem upon an artfully constructed mask. The result is *self-image-esteem* which is different than self-esteem. Even talented, wealthy, successful people remain restless, anxious, and insecure if they hide behind a social mask. We find self esteem through authenticity and self-compassion, which comes when we see and accept both our light and our shadow. Embracing the shadow is one of the most powerful shifts a human being can make.

You are unable to become yourself, or even accept yourself, until you know yourself. Once you know, accept, and become yourself, you accept and live in harmony with others in your world.

As you come to accept yourself as you are, you will discover the compassion to accept your partner, parents, children, and friends **as they are**. The world becomes a 'come as you are' party.

Paradoxically, as you embrace your shadow and your world, this acceptance opens the way to positive change. You come to realize how exhausting your social facade can be. With that realization, life becomes a relaxed opportunity for growth, instead of a flight from inferiority; you continue to improve without having anything to prove. You become more of who you are.

What we as humans perceive as reality is a dance of dualities - night and day, light and darkness, high and low. Of course, it is far more pleasant to contemplate our light, our hopes and dreams, than to explore our dark side. So why open Pandora's box if there are parts of yourself you dislike? Why acknowledge and investigate them? Since your shadow is, by definition, what you would rather keep hidden and unacknowledged, the idea of embracing it may seem like a task you would rather do later. Much later.

Light has always been more popular than shadow. Even though 'Illuminating Your Shadow' is one of the less pleasant areas to explore, it may ultimately be one of the most transformational, leading to self-knowledge, compassion, forgiveness, freedom, and authenticity. The reasons for embracing, accepting, and illuminating your darker side are many

There is no need to deny or repress parts of us that are dishonest, unkind or 'bad' in order to be 'good'. We only need to avoid animating them and instead heal, transmute and release them, while integrating the positive transmuted parts.

We leave *Illuminate Your Shadow* by revisiting the issue of self-worth. This is relevant here, because exploring your shadow, tends to lower your sense of self-worth to the degree it was based upon an illusory, self-serving self-image. At the same time, this process provides a more complete, balanced, realistic view of our conduct and relations with others. Ultimately it's a great relief to finally realize that I'm **not** okay, and you're **not** okay, and that's okay.

Illuminating your shadow reveals that there is no need to deserve life's blessings by virtue of having earned them with all your good works, and that Spirit continually supports and blesses you. Whether you happen to *feel* deserving or undeserving becomes irrelevant. The sun and the air and the song of the bird, the support and love of family or friends, remain. The blessings of Spirit shower upon you in a hundred forms each day. This is more than merely a sentimental platitude, and is a moment to moment reality you notice when your attention is free to do so.

Having seen yourself as you are, accepted both your light and shadow, you will find that your dependence on a *feeling* of self-worth is replaced by a reliance on and acceptance of the innate and unconditional worth of all reality, which includes all creatures, things, and people, *and* you. In finding your own wholeness, you transcend the need for self-worth and simply become willing to accept life's blessings and opportunities no matter what your *feelings* in regards to 'worthiness.

The fact is, sometimes we act kindly and sometimes callously, sometimes honestly and sometimes less so, sometimes we are givers, sometimes takers. Illuminating your shadow, you find compassion for the foibles, illusions, and shadows of yourself and others.

Illuminate Your Shadow - Statements/Questions	Best If	Before Clearing	After Clearing
If someone offends me, calls me a name, or accuses me of something, do I automatically defend myself?	NO		
Do I *feel* resentful when I give more than I receive?	NO		
Do I know my self's fears?	YES		
Have I illuminated my shadow as is best at this time?	YES		
Have I explored beneath the veneer of my personality and self image as is best at this time?	YES		
Have I LOVED and accepted my shadow as a part of me?	YES		
Have I transcended the need for self-worth and am I simply willing to accept life's blessings and opportunities no matter what my *feelings* of self-worth?	YES		
Have I ever stolen or lied? Unless you are a saint the answer is yes			
Have I forgiven myself, my-self and my-Self for past lies or thefts?	YES		
Name two or three of other people's traits or behaviors that bother me the most. 1 ( ) 2 ( ) 3 ( )			
Is there a part of me that would like to behave that way?			
Repeat the same questions using your full birth name and any other name you go by instead of 'I'			

10 - Sexuality And Sensuality

Now, having opened the door to your personal shadow, you are ready to embrace and illuminate the shadows of your sexuality.

Enlightened sexuality has less to do with your skills of foreplay than your capacity for intimacy, your communion with Spirit through the arms of your lover and joy in every aspect of your life.

Shame, guilt and embarrassment are unknown to us until we learn such *feelings* from our parents or others who socialize us in much the same way they were socialized.

Whatever faith we practice, if any, we need to realize that sexuality has no inherent morality or immorality. Such ideas are a human invention.

Sexuality and Sensuality - Statements/Questions	Best If	Before Clearing	After Clearing
Do I judge my own or other's fantasies as 'wrong'?	NO		
Am I ashamed of my negative/destructive fantasies?	NO		
Do I judge those who choose a hedonistic path?	NO		
Do I judge those who choose a puritanical path?	NO		
Do I fully accept myself as I am?	YES		
Do I love myself.?	YES		
Have I embraced myself as I am and released all judgments about my perceived lack of perfection?	YES		
Have I embraced my soul's and body's sensuality.?	YES		
Have I unified both hemispheres of my brain and transcended my gender role so I can animate at will both masculine and feminine qualities?	YES		
Am I capable of hardness or softness and am I able to turn outward or inward?	YES		
Am I whole, and even though I am physically male or female, my character and qualities have evolved to a state of inclusive androgyny. (Inclusive androgyny entails the ability to access and embody both masculine and feminine qualities and capacities.)	YES		
Am I unconditionally LOVING and accepting of my fantasies?	YES		
Have I found and embraced a balance between self-denial (puritanical) and self-indulgence (hedonistic) tendencies? (Remember neither is superior to the other)	YES		
Do I sense and accept the value of either self-denial or self-indulgence depending on the situation?	YES		
Am I aware of my puritanical and hedonistic aspects?	YES		
Have I balanced and reconciled my puritanical and hedonistic aspects?	YES		
Have I embraced and integrated my spirituality and sexuality?	YES		
Have I balanced my use of sensory experience under the dominion of my higher -self?	YES		
As I recognize my fantasies do I heal and release them with LOVE and without judgment?	YES		
Repeat the same questions using your full birth name and any other name you go by instead of 'I'			

11 - Awaken And Open Your Heart

No one can teach Love or learn it, for the mind has no heart and the heart has no reason.

Self love is a beginning practice of Love. You need to Love yourself before you can truly Love another - a parent, a pet, a friend, a partner, the larger world.

As you master the will to act Loving - to show kindness and compassion in any moment despite *feelings* to the contrary - you develop the capacity to give unconditional Love. If your spouse, child, friend, partner or even a stranger is yelling at you or blaming you, you are unlikely to *feel* love and compassion for them in the moment; still you never lose the power to act with kindness.

Allow your attention to rise into the heart so you naturally speak, think, hear, touch and act from the heart.

Listen from your heart and you will automatically listen without judgment, expectations or opinions.

The simple, pleasurable practices of connecting your heart to your voice, thought, sight, touch and hearing are forms of spiritual practice that produces emotional healing in relationships. Regardless of the impact or lack of impact you notice on others, you will soon know their impact on your awakening heart.

Awaken and Open Your Heart - Statements/Questions	Best If	Before Clearing	After Clearing
Am I willing to risk the pain and sorrow of loss?	YES		
Do I trust myself enough to open my heart to joy?	YES		
Do I know there is no safety in love and none is needed?	YES		
Has my attention risen to the level of LOVE and service, and to the mystical levels beyond? (Some people call this the level of the heart or fourth chakra.)	YES		
Have I opened my heart to love and to LOVE?	YES		
Repeat the same questions using your full birth name and any other name you go by instead of 'I'			

12 – Serve Your World And Your Self

We begin "Serving Our World" by resolving the apparent contradiction between healing ('working on') ones-self and serving others.

Serve Your World and Your Self - Statements/Questions	Best If	Before Clearing	After Clearing
When I do something for someone do I expect thanks?	NO		
Does a part of me *feel* I need to do healing, transmuting, releasing and integrating for others?	NO		
Have I resolved, for myself, the apparent contradiction between serving myself and serving others?	YES		
When I do something for someone is it possible I should be the one thanking them?	YES		
Do I know and am I aware that I do all healing, transmuting, releasing and integrating for myself even when assisting others.	YES		
Am I combining my unique talents and abilities to serve LOVE?	YES		
Do I have passion for what I do and am I expressing/sharing my unique talents and gifts as is best?	YES		
Do I ask, "How can I help/assist?" instead of "What is in it for me?"	YES		
Do I ask for all guidance to come from my "Higher Self" and Great Spirit/God and that I understand the guidance clearly and as is best?	YES		
What are my unique talents and abilities? ( )			
What am here to give and share? ( )			
How can I best serve? ( )			
How am I best suited to serve humanity? ( )			
Repeat the same questions using your full birth name and any other name you go by instead of 'I'			

The practices above are a process, an ongoing journey, rather than a destination. Adapted by author from *Everyday Enlightenment - The Twelve Gateways to Personal Growth* by Dan Millman

Other Thoughts To Ponder

Am I here to contact my higher self or to become my higher self?
What do I really want to do with my life?
What are my definitions of success? (health, wealth, wisdom, power and prestige, well-being, joy)
Do I value information (data) or intuition and wisdom more?
Do I set aside at least five or ten minutes each day for quiet time?
Do I turn off my cell phone, TV, stereo, radio, tablet, computer and email and truly disconnect from distractions for at least a few minutes per day?
Do I slow down enough to search my soul?
Do I **react** with fear and anger or do I **act** with Love and compassion?
Does anger, hate and violence breed and attract anger, hate and violence?
Does Love and compassion breed and attract Love and compassion?
Are 'primitive' societies that are filled with joy and peace with a close connection to nature really primitive? Are they actually more advanced than 'civilized' societies?

Chapter 14
Tools, Crutches and Traps

All tools when used as a key to open to the next level are useful and in harmony with life and Great Spirit. When the next level is reached let go of the old tool. It may be replaced with a new tool or level of awareness.

Almost anything can be used as a tool. This includes, Drums, rattles, stones, crystals, 'Crystal Skulls, 'Sacred Pipes', candles, incense, dragons blood, sage, sweet-grass, meditation pillows, mantras repeated over and over out loud or silently, astrology, numerology, sacred ceremony etc.

When you reach for one of these tools or sacred items, if you hear a gentle and LOVING voice, saying something like, "Please, you do**n't** need that, for you have all that you need inside of you", it may be time to let go of the perceived need of the item. Realize that it is Great Spirit within and without that gives these items their ability to assist you.

You need no sacred external things. Sacred things are **but** triggers to your consciousness, outward expressions of inward realities. Sacred objects are powerful in and of themselves, **but** at best they are tools to help carry you to spiritual consciousness. They are a camouflage for the masses, a trigger for young spiritual searchers, and are a crutch for those who refuse to let them go. Once you have used a spiritual object and understand its power, you must learn to get to that power from within, rather than with an external crutch, otherwise the object becomes a self-limiting crutch. These objects you will always hold in reverence. As your power grows and you learn to tap these same powers from within, there is no need for the symbol or sacred object. You can then leave them home or pass them on to assist others to grow. Sometimes you may find yourself using them for the benefit of others who still require an outward sign.

Even mantras repeated over and over silently or out load, meditation pillows, astrology and numerology are really nothing more than tools. Let go of them when you realize they no longer serve your highest purpose and have become crutches and traps.

Sacred Ceremony is also a tool. It is really the heart filled with LOVE that makes the connection to Great Spirit/Divinity.

When you can meditate without a meditation pillow or special position let them go and pass them on or put them aside.

If you use a tool because you enjoy it, keep using it with awareness that it is really Great Spirit and your intent, thoughts and beliefs that are the real tools. If you use it because you think you have to, is it a tool, crutch or trap?

Also, be aware that tools can be used for and with LOVE or for and with energies that are selfish fear based or of ego.

Even prescription and natural medicines and supplements are tools. So is surgery. Use them as long as there is a perceived need for them. Let go of them only when there is no longer a perceived need and you can maintain your health without them. As an example, I developed a major, life threatening, infection in 1981 after abdominal surgery and a very serious jaw infection in 1997. I was on intravenous antibiotics for almost two weeks in 1981 and prescription antibiotics in 1997. The surgeries and antibiotics saved my life and gave me time to continue my life's journey.

If I get an infection I use, grapefruit seed extract, olive leaf extract and other natural remedies in place of prescription antibiotics. Be aware there are medicines, herbs and supplements that interfere with each other and can be dangerous when used together. As an example, if you are taking a prescription blood thinner or one for high blood pressure eating grapefruit could be very dangerous. Since Grapefruit Seed Extract comes from grapefruit it may be dangerous too. The improper combination of herbs and other natural substances can also be dangerous. Be sure you know what you are doing or consult an expert.

If I had a serious enough infection or injury I would still use ALL methods available as I *felt* appropriate.

Be aware that **not** all vitamins are natural. As an example vitamin E can be synthetic and man-made or it can be extracted in its natural form from plants. There is evidence that synthetic vitamins and medicines are less helpful than the natural counterpart, and may even be harmful. Organic spinach is healthy for almost everyone, however with its high purine content it can worsen or even bring on gout.

As a child from about five to 9 years old I ran around in circles to either quiet my mind or keep other thoughts out. When that was no longer socially acceptable I played football or basketball almost every day. There was almost always a pickup game I could find and I played the entire game. When I was in tenth or eleventh grade I broke my right ankle badly. I was confined to bed for about two weeks and had no way to quiet my mind and keep other's thoughts out. I started smoking. I have smoked since then except for two six-month stretches when I was involved with outside activities that I truly enjoyed and kept my mind occupied. I know these were tools and or crutches. Smoking may have kept me from being overwhelmed and may have kept me off mind numbing prescription drugs up to now. I feel it is now a crutch and a trap. It is time to quiet my mind myself knowing that the ability, Spirit and answer is within and there is no need to run in circles, smoke or use any other inward or outward crutch or tool.

Books, including this one, can be tools, crutches or traps. The answers and abilities really come from within.

Suggested Reading And Web Sites

My First Book and Web Site

Two Choices - Divine Love or Anything Else by Glenn Molinari

http://twochoices.net   for additional information and FREE PDFs

Dental And Mouth

Elements of Danger: Protect Yourself Against the Hazards of Modern Dentistry by Morton Walker, D.P.M. (can be overwhelming)

<http://www.hugginsappliedhealing.com/>

<http://www.talkinternational.com/toothchart.html> (for interactive tooth to organ chart)

<http://www.flcv.com/indexa.html>

<http://www.secretofthieves.com/tooth-chart/> (an even more detailed tooth to organ chart)

Nutrition

No one nutritional and eating plan is right for everyone. When looked at with a critical eye the following three plans combine for a good basis.

Eat Right For Your Type by Dr. Peter J. D'Adamo

    <http://dadamo.com/>
Enter The Zone by Barry Sears, PhD

    <http://zonediet.com/zone-diet-overview>
The Metabolic Typing Diet by William Wolcott and Trish Fahey

    <http://www.healthexcel.com/>
<http:/FindaSpring.com> (can help you find a natural spring close to you)

Affirmations

You Can Heal Your Life by Louise L. Hay

Memories Replaying

Zero Limits by Ihaleakala Hew Len, PhD and Joe Vitale

A very good introduction to healing and releasing Memories Replaying. by practicing Self Identity Ho'oponopono as developed and taught by Morrnah Nalamaku Simeona and Ihaleakala Hew Len. I have been unable to find a web site that is Ihaleakala Hew Lens'. His teachings are very powerful, however many people have commercialized them.

<http://top411.tripod.com/zero-limits-with-hooponopono/dr_ihaleakala_hew_len.html>

(A web page with links to video interviews with Ihaleakala Hew Len)

Trapped/Hidden Feelings, Emotions and Aspects

The Emotion Code by Dr. Bradley Nelson

<http://www.drbradleynelson.com/filters/the-emotion-code/>

Emotional Clearing Process by John Ruskan

<http://www.emclear.com/index.html>\

The Dark Side Of The Light Chasers by Debbie Ford

<http://store.debbieford.com/product_info.php?products_id=9>

Magnets For Healing

<https://www.lyonlegacy.com/learn/behind_science_magnetics.aspx>

The Ringing Cedars Series by Vladimir Megre

This series of books tells of Vladimir's learning from a Siberian recluse named Anastasia.

Some people believe Vladimir Megre has met Anastasia and the book is based on actual events. Some People say it is a work of fiction. Some people even say that there is no such person as Vladimir Megre.

I just found a web site <http://archive.org/advancedsearch.php> that has all 9 books in the series available as FREE downloads in EPUB, MOBI for Kindle and PDF formats. The PDF with text is searchable for words and phrases.

Book 1 *Anastasia* by Vladimir Megre

Book 2 *The Ringing Cedars of Russia* by Vladimir Megre

Book 3 *The Space of Love* by Vladimir Megre

Book 4 *Co-Creation* by Vladimir Megre

Book 5 *Who Are We?* by Vladimir Megre

Book 6 *The Book Of Kin* by Vladimir Megre

Book 7 *The Energy of Life* by Vladimir Megre

Book 8.1 *The New Civilization* by Vladimir Megre

Book 8.2 *Rites of Love* by Vladimir Megre

<http://www.vladimirmegre.com/vladimir_megre_story.php>

<http://www.anastasia.ca/>

Good information on Muscle testing

<http://www.holistichealthtools.com/muscle.html>

Excellent Practice (modify for yourself)

Everyday Enlightenment - The Twelve Gateways to Personal Growth by Dan Millman

References

Books

D'Adamo, Peter. (1996). *Eat Right For Your Type*. New York: G. P. Putnam's & Sons.

Hay, Louise. (2004). *You Can Heal Your Life*. Hay House, Inc.

Hew Len, Ihaleakala, & Vitale, Joe. (2007). *Zero Limits*. Hoboken, New Jersey: John Wiley & Sons.

McKenna, Jed. (2007). *Spiritual Warfare*. WiseFool Press

Megre, Vladimir. (1996). *Anastasia*. Ed. Leonid Sharashkin. Trans. John Woodsworth. The Ringing Cedars Series. Book 1. Ringing Cedars Press. Kahului, HI.

Megre, Vladimir. (1997). *The Ringing Cedars Of Russia*. Ed. Leonid Sharashkin. Trans. John Woodsworth. The Ringing Cedars Series. Book 2. Ringing Cedars Press. Kahului, HI.

Megre, Vladimir. (1998). *The Space of Love*. Ed. Leonid Sharashkin. Trans. John Woodsworth. The Ringing Cedars Series. Book 3. Ringing Cedars Press. Kahului, HI.

Megre, Vladimir. (2000). *Co-Creation*. Ed. Leonid Sharashkin. Trans. John Woodsworth. The Ringing Cedars Series. Book 4. Kahului, HI. Ringing Cedars Press.

Megre, Vladimir. (2001). *Who Are We*. Ed. Leonid Sharashkin. Trans. John Woodsworth. The Ringing Cedars Series. Book 5. Kahului, HI. Ringing Cedars Press.

Megre, Vladimir. (2002). *The Book Of Kin*. Ed. Leonid Sharashkin. Trans. John Woodsworth. The Ringing Cedars Series. Book 6. Kahului, HI. Ringing Cedars Press.

Megre, Vladimir. (2003). *The Energy Of Life*. Ed. Leonid Sharashkin. Trans. John Woodsworth. The Ringing Cedars Series. Book 7. Kahului, HI. Ringing Cedars Press.

Megre, Vladimir. (2005). *The New Civilization*. Ed. Leonid Sharashkin. Trans. John Woodsworth. The Ringing Cedars Series. Book 8.1. Kahului, HI. Ringing Cedars Press.

Megre, Vladimir. (2006). *Rites Of Love*. Ed. Leonid Sharashkin. Trans. John Woodsworth. The Ringing Cedars Series. Book 8.2. Kahului, HI. Ringing Cedars Press.

Millman, Dan. (1998). *Everyday Enlightenment : the twelve gateways to personal growth*. New York: Warner Books Inc.

Nelson, Bradley. (2007). *The Emotion Code*. Mesquite, Nevada: Wellness Unmasked.

Ruskan, John. (2003). *Emotional Clearing: An East/West Guide to Releasing Negative Feelings* and Awakening Unconditional Happiness. New York: R. Wyler& Co.

Sears, Barry. (1995). *Enter The Zone*. New York: Harper Collins.

Summer Rain, Mary. (1990). *Earthway*. New York: Pocket Books.

Walker, Morton. (2000). *Elements of Danger*. Charlottesville, Virginia: Hampton Roads.

Whitaker, Kay C. (1991). *The Reluctant Shaman. A Woman's First Encounters with the Unseen Spirits Of The Earth*. New York: Harper Collins.

Wolcott, William. (2002). *The Metabolic Typing Diet*. New York: Broadway Books.

Web Sites

Babcock, Brent. (n.d.). *Vanishing Twins*. Retrieved December, 16 2013, from
http://www.vanishingtwin.com/index.php/main-menu-definition

Bernardi, Kathleen. (n.d.). *Woodland Dental Hygiene.* Retrieved February, 8 2014, from
http://woodlanddental.ca/press/2010/08/31/history-of-mercury-amalgam/

Bernardi, Kathleen. (n.d.). *Woodland Dental Hygiene.* Retrieved February, 8 2014, from
http://woodlanddental.ca/press/2010/09/14/banning-elemental-mercury-in-amalgam-fillings/

Bernardi, Kathleen. (n.d.). *Woodland Dental Hygiene.* Retrieved February, 8 2014, from
http://woodlanddental.ca/press/2010/09/22/waging-war-on-mercury-amalgam-fillings/

Bernardi, Kathleen. (n.d.). *Woodland Dental Hygiene.* Retrieved February, 8 2014, from
http://woodlanddental.ca/press/2010/10/06/should-you-consider-having-your-mercury-amalgam-fillings-removed/

Bernardi, Kathleen. (n.d.). *Woodland Dental Hygiene.* Retrieved February, 8 2014, from
http://woodlanddental.ca/press/2010/10/14/removing-mercury-amalgam-fillings/

Bernardi, Kathleen. (n.d.). *Woodland Dental Hygiene.* Retrieved February, 8 2014, from
http://woodlanddental.ca/press/2010/12/16/fda-revisits-the-safety-of-dental-amalgam/

Dennis, Caryl. (n.d.). *Rainbows Unlimited*. Retrieved December, 16 2013, from
http://caryl.ipower.com/wordpress/vanishing-twins/

Florida League of Conservation Voters Education Fund. *Incidence
Levels and Chronic Health Effects Related to Cavitations.*
Retrieved December, 17 2013 from http://www.flcv.com/cavitati.html

Lee, John, M.D. and Hopkins, Virginia. (n.d.). *Xenohormones (Part I) and Your Health.*
Retrieved December, 16 2013, from
http://www.virginiahopkinstestkits.com/xenohormoneI.html

Lee, John, M.D. and Hopkins, Virginia. (n.d.). *Xenohormones (Part II) in Your
Environment.* Retrieved December, 16, 2013, from
http://www.virginiahopkinstestkits.com/xenohormoneII.html

Lilypad Productions Trust. *Thieves oil blend - Arm yourself with the power of Thieves.*
Retrieved December, 17 2013 from http://www.secretofthieves.com/tooth-chart/index.cfm

Mercola, Dr Joseph. (n.d.). *Take Control Of Your Health.* Retrieved December, 16 2013,
from http://articles.mercola.com/sites/articles/archive/2010/09/11/alkaline-water-interview.aspx

Oasis Advanced Wellness. Retrieved December, 17 2013, from
http://www.oasisadvancedwellness.com/tools/tooth-chart-top.htm#01

Oasis Advanced Wellness. Retrieved December, 17 2013, from
http://www.oasisadvancedwellness.com/tools/tooth-chart-btm.htm#17

Warren, Charlotte and Cummins, Ronnie. *GMO Grass: Coming to a Lawn Near You?*
Retrieved June, 1 2014, from http://gmofreeplanet.com/uncategorized/
gmo-grass-coming-lawn-near

Women Living Naturally. *Xenohormones and xenoestrogens.*
Retrieved December, 16 2013, from http://www.womenlivingnaturally.com/
articlepage.php?id=73

Seminars

Hew Len, Ihaleakala. *Self I-dentity through Ho'oponopono Basic.* IZI LLC.
Woodland Hills, CA. Oct 31 and November 1, 2009

About The Author

Glenn Molinari was born in Wilmington, Delaware on April 17, 1948. Until 1954, his family lived in Southern New Jersey, at which time the family moved to the suburbs just outside Wilmington. Glenn served our Country in the Air Force from 1968 to 1972. After having been honorably discharged, he moved back to Delaware and in 1996 moved in with his father on the Eastern Shore of Maryland.

In 1997, Glenn became involved with alternative medicine to address personal health issues that Western Medicine had been unable to diagnose or to cure. While Glenn was learning about alternative therapies and the Body/Mind/Spirit connections, he remained at his father's side as caregiver until 2007. He moved to Cornville, Arizona in 2008, where he resides today.

Glenn continues his interest in alternative healing modalities and has made many Spiritual connections in Sedona, AZ through his interests.

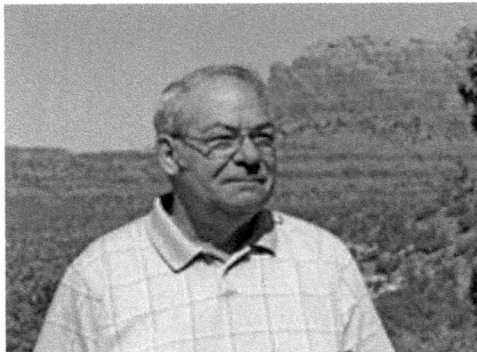

I hope you have found this helpful.

If you wish, you may contact Glenn Molinari

telephone: 1 (928) 300-6202

email: glenn@twoChoices.net

Web Site: http://twoChoices.net

www.ingramcontent.com/pod-product-compliance
Lightning Source LLC
Chambersburg PA
CBHW081654270326
41933CB00017B/3161